# BASIC HEALTH PUBLICATIONS
## USER'S GUIDE

# TO

# VITAMIN C

*Learn What You Need to Know about How Vitamin C Can Improve Your Total Health.*

## HYLA CASS, M.D. & JIM ENGLISH
JACK CHALLEM Series Editor

The information contained in this book is based upon the research and personal and professional experiences of the authors. It is not intended as a substitute for consulting with your physician or other healthcare provider. Any attempt to diagnose and treat an illness should be done under the direction of a healthcare professional.

The publisher does not advocate the use of any particular healthcare protocol but believes the information in this book should be available to the public. The publisher and authors are not responsible for any adverse effects or consequences resulting from the use of the suggestions, preparations, or procedures discussed in this book. Should the reader have any questions concerning the appropriateness of any procedures or preparation mentioned, the authors and the publisher strongly suggest consulting a professional healthcare advisor.

Series Editor: Jack Challem
Editor: Carol Rosenberg
Typesetter: Gary A. Rosenberg
Series Cover Designer: Mike Stromberg

Basic Health Publications User's Guides are published by Basic Health Publications, Inc.
8200 Boulevard East
North Bergen, NJ 07047
1-800-575-8890

Printed in the United States of America

10 9 8 7 6 5 4 3 2 1

# CONTENTS

# INTRODUCTION

Today, vitamin C is one of the most widely used and highly valued vitamins in the world—and for good reason. Its popularity began in 1970, when Linus Pauling published his groundbreaking book *Vitamin C and the Common Cold*. Sales of vitamin C immediately skyrocketed, with some amazing results, such as the number of deaths attributed to heart disease plummeting by a staggering 40 percent in the next decade. Scientist now estimate that more than 250,000 lives are saved every year because of the efforts of Linus Pauling and other dedicated researchers to educate the public about the benefits of vitamin C. Based on these statistics, it has been estimated that if everyone in the United States took several hundred milligrams of vitamin C a day, more than 100,000 lives and $100 billion in healthcare costs would be saved each year.

In *The Users Guide to Vitamin C*, we will show you how vitamin C reduces heart disease, cancer, and many of the common diseases that plague the world today. We will also look at how a genetic accident that occurred untold millions of years ago robbed our ancestors of the ability to manufacture this vital nutrient. This problem has continued to trouble humankind throughout history, and even today, it contributes to the vast majority of human diseases, such as arthritis, cardiovascular disease, strokes, and cancer. We will see that these conditions, which are so common in humans, rarely occur in animals that still possess the ability to manufacture vitamin C—often in amounts thousands of times greater than those many health authorities consider to be essential to human health.

Not only can vitamin C help us to feel better and live longer, but it also has been proven to support numerous functions that can help us attain optimal health, including:

- Antioxidant Protection. This premier antioxidant nutrient protects us from the ravages of free radicals that, if left to destroy cell membranes and damage DNA, lead to the development of degenerative diseases and accelerated aging.

- Collagen Production. Vitamin C helps manufacture collagen, the basic cellular "cement" that keeps muscles, tendons, bones, teeth, and skin healthy and strong, and aids in the repair of blood vessels and broken bones.

- Cardiovascular Support. Vitamin C benefits heart conditions of all kinds, normalizes blood pressure, reduces cholesterol levels, and aids in the removal of cholesterol deposits from arterial walls.

In the following chapters, you will also see how a nutrient that is so abundant in nature—and so necessary for all life—is constantly under attack from those who argue that all good nutrition begins and ends with a fork. Can we get all the vitamin C we need from food alone? It has been shown that even the best diet cannot begin to provide the higher levels of vitamin C (500–1,000 mg per day) that research has proven can help us fend off illness, degenerative diseases, and premature aging.

We will also address the safety of vitamin C—an issue that is often at the center of seemingly biased media reporting that ignores the overwhelming body of clinical and scientific research that attests to the safety and effectiveness of this natural nutrient.

So we invite you to sit back, pour a glass of orange juice (or take a good multivitamin), and come along to discover how this essential anti-aging, anticancer, and antistress nutrient can help you live a longer, healthier, and more fulfilling life.

# CHAPTER 1

# THE HISTORY
# OF VITAMIN C
# AND SCURVY

**V**itamin C, also called ascorbic acid, is a powerful water-soluble antioxidant that is vital for the growth and maintenance of all body tissues. Though easily absorbed by the intestines, vitamin C cannot be stored in the body, and is excreted in the urine within two to four hours of ingestion. Human history has been deeply influenced by vitamin C—or more accurately, by a frequent and disastrous lack of this vital nutrient. In his book *The Healing Factor: Vitamin C Against Disease,* the late biochemist Irwin Stone stated: ". . . the lack of this molecule [vitamin C] in humans has contributed to more deaths, sickness, and just plain misery than any other single factor in man's long history."

Written records dating back to ancient Egypt contain the earliest reports of scurvy, a dreaded human disease caused by vitamin C deficiency. In 450 B.C., Aristotle carefully described the symptoms of scurvy, which include muscle weakness, lethargy, extreme fatigue, depression, joint pains, swollen and bleeding gums, foul breath, loss of teeth, bleeding under the skin and orifices (hemorrhages), and, eventually, death.

**Ascorbic Acid**
*Another name for vitamin C that derives from the Latin word* ascorbic, *which means "without scurvy."*

Scurvy has remained a constant threat to humans, causing death and misery whenever dietary

sources of vitamin C became scarce. Outbreaks
have been particularly devastating in times of extreme famine, such as during the Irish Potato
Famine. And throughout history, scurvy often has
been more dangerous than man-made weapons,
decimating entire armies cut off from supplies of
fresh fruits and vegetables. During the Crusades
(1200 A.D.), untold thousands perished from
scurvy, as did hundreds of thousands of soldiers
fighting in the Crimean, Napoleonic, and American
Civil wars.

Outbreaks of scurvy have not been restricted
just to the land. In the sixteenths century, the Re-
naissance saw the introduction of modern seafaring
and a subsequent rush for global exploration. During this period, scurvy became the dreaded
scourge of the sea, as sailors embarked on epic
voyages that often lasted for two years or more.
Frequently, captains would return from a voyage
with barely a third of their crews still desperately
clinging to life. Such appalling losses of life (and
money) were unacceptable to European ambitions,
and led to a desperate search for a cure for scurvy.

## Dr. James Lind and the
## Birth of the "Limey"

In 1739, England was entering into a war with
Spain. In a daring tactical move, the British Navy
dispatched a fleet of ships to the Philippines to attack the famed Manila galleons that plied riches,
men, and supplies between Manila, Mexico, and
South America in support of the Spanish colonial
empire. In 1740, under the command of British
Admiral Anson, six ships and 1,100 men departed
England. After circumnavigating the world, Admiral Anson returned four years later with thirty-two
wagons of Spanish treasure, but at a terrible cost
of life. He had lost almost 90 percent of his men

to scurvy and, in the end, could barely muster enough men to help sail the last surviving ship back to England.

One of the survivors of Anson's epic voyage was a Scottish naval surgeon named James Lind, who returned from the trip a deeply shaken man. Appalled by the pain, suffering, and loss of life he witnessed on the ships, he was dedicated to finding a cure for scurvy. In 1746, Lind began to study the disease, taking pains to monitor the diet and health of sailors, while carefully tracking the progression of symptoms. In his book *A Treatise on Scurvy,* Lind described his observations aboard the *H.M.S. Salisbury:* "Scurvy began to rage after being a month or six weeks at sea . . . the water on board . . . was uncommonly sweet and good [and] provisions such as could afford no suspicion . . . yet, at the expiration of ten weeks, we brought into Plymouth 80 men, out of a complement of 350, more or less afflicted with the diseases."

Since the ships of Lind's time lacked modern refrigeration, sailors on long voyages lived on a diet composed of nonperishable foods, such as grains, beans, and dried bread. Lind suspected that the cause of scurvy was related to the absence of some dietary factor, other than carbohydrates, fat, and protein. To test his theory, Lind conducted an experiment during a ten-week sea voyage.

Lind first selected twelve sailors showing signs of scurvy, and divided them into six groups of two men each. During the course of the voyage, Lind gave each pair an experimental substance in addition to their basic shipboard diet. Every day each pair received either a quart of cider, an elixir containing sulfuric acid, seawater, a combination of mustard and horseradish, a spoonful of vinegar, or two oranges and one lemon.

Four of the groups showed no improvement,

while the pair receiving the cider reported slight improvement of their symptoms. Most impressive was the response of the two men who were given oranges and lemons: they completely recovered from all of their symptoms. In this manner, Lind is credited with establishing that the addition of citrus fruits would effectively prevent scurvy.

He published his findings in his 1753 landmark *A Treatise on Scurvy*. Unfortunately, his discovery was largely ignored for another forty years, during which time another 100,000 British sailors died from scurvy. Eventually, the British Navy issued orders for all ships to carry lemons and limes for the sailors to consume on a daily basis. Among citrus fruits, limes from the British West Indies were especially abundant, and their frequent appearance on British ships earned English sailors the lasting, if not appreciated, nickname "limeys."

## The Discovery of Vitamin C (Ascorbic Acid)

Even though Lind had proven that the missing nutrient that led to scurvy was contained in citrus fruits (as well as potatoes, sauerkraut, rose hips, and other plants), the exact nature of this vital nutrient continued to puzzle scientists for the next two centuries.

The first breakthrough in vitamin C research occurred in 1926, when the Hungarian scientist Albert Szent-Györgyi, M.D., Ph.D., traveled to Cambridge University to conduct research on the chemical processes that caused fruits and vegetables to turn brown. Szent-Györgyi first succeeded in isolating a white crystalline substance from the adrenal gland of cows, which he referred to as Cx11.

Later, in 1928, Szent-Györgyi isolated these same crystals from the juice of potatoes and cabbages, and renamed the substance hexuronic acid.

Szent-Györgyi later collaborated with the famed English chemist W. Haworth, and together they finally determined the chemical structure of hexuronic acid ($C_6H_8O_6$). Finally, in 1932, after producing the first pure crystals of vitamin C, Szent-Györgyi and Haworth once again renamed the substance, and, in recognition of its role in preventing scurvy, called it ascorbic acid, from the Latin word *ascorbic,* which means "without scurvy."

Five years later, in 1937, Szent-Györgyi was awarded the Nobel Prize in Medicine "for his discoveries in connection with the biological combustion processes, with special reference to vitamin C and the catalysis of fumaric acid."

## The Missing Link—Unraveling the Secrets of Vitamin C

Following the groundbreaking work of Szent-Györgyi, researchers began to slowly unravel the structure and chemistry of vitamin C. They discovered that vitamin C is a carbohydrate closely related to glucose, the simple sugar that is used by most living organisms as a fuel for cellular energy. They also learned that most plants and animals possess an enzyme called gluconolactone oxidase (or GLO for short) that allows them to readily convert glucose into vitamin C.

Next, researchers made one of the most startling findings of all—that somehow humans had lost the ability to do what virtually every other form of life on earth can do with ease—to manufacture vitamin C. This inability, which is shared with only a few other mammals, such as apes and guinea pigs, set the stage for more research as scientists struggled to understand how humans could have lost the ability to manufacture something that is so necessary for life and so easily produced by other all other living organisms. What happened, why did it happen, and what did it mean in terms of human health?

## From Sugar to Vitamin C

In order to understand the importance of vitamin C and its vital role in virtually every life form, we need to momentarily gaze back through time to

**Enzymes**
*Protein structures that act as catalysts to promote the billions of biochemical reactions necessary for virtually all life processes.*

the earliest moments of life on earth. Scientists now know that the ability to synthesize vitamin C was a trait acquired early in the development of life. Billions of years ago, the earth's atmosphere was rich in carbon dioxide and contained only minute amounts of oxygen. In order to survive in such a hostile environment, the earliest living organisms eventually learned to "capture" or scavenge rare oxygen electrons from the environment. This new adaptation not only aided the survival of these early life forms, but it also contributed to another giant leap in early evolution—the development of plant photosynthesis.

Photosynthesis, in turn, removed carbon dioxide and increased oxygen levels in the atmosphere over a period of billions of years. By radically altering the atmosphere, this process also led to the evolution of complex multicellular life forms that were totally dependent on oxygen. Interestingly, one type of life that did not acquire the ability to synthesize vitamin C was primitive, single-celled organisms that are still alive today—bacteria. This is an important point that explains why vitamin C is so effective against certain forms of bacteria. The result of this early reliance on vitamin C for scavenging electrons is that every form of life on earth today (except for anaerobic bacteria) needs vitamin C, whether they can synthesize it or not.

## The "Lost" Enzyme

All life on earth was originally endowed with the ability to manufacture vitamin C from the simple sugar, glucose. Today, almost all plants produce vitamin C. Some, such as strawberries, rose hips, green peppers, and citrus fruit, produce it in relatively large amounts. Almost all animals have retained their ability to generate vitamin C in the liver, usually in amounts much higher than those that could be obtained from dietary sources. For example, a goat, weighing as much as an average man, produces 13 g of vitamin C each day—more than two hundred times the current human recommended daily allowance (RDA) of 90 mg per day. And other animals, including dogs, mice, and even elephants, also produce vitamin C in amounts that, relative to their body weight, would be the equivalent of a human taking 10 g of vitamin C every day!

At some point in the early development of life, our ancestors lost the ability to synthesize vitamin C. Scientists believe this change occurred between 45 and 60 million years ago. Some believe that early members of the primate family somehow lost the use of a gene that the body needs to produce vitamin C. The loss of this functioning gene may have been caused by random genetic mutation. Another theory proposes that the gene was actually damaged by free radicals or by an attack by a virus.

Some scientists now believe that the loss of this functioning gene was actually a beneficial change that helped our species adapt and evolve. One proposed advantage was, that by getting their vitamin C from food, our early ancestors were able to use more glucose for energy production, giving them an adaptive advantage over other species. Additionally, it has been proposed that the increased production of free radicals that resulted from the loss of this gene contributed to a greater number of genetic mutations that played a role in the evolution of higher primates, including humans.

It was only when our early humanoid ancestors began to leave the vitamin C–rich habitats, such as the jungles and rainforests, that the true nature of the loss became apparent in the form of new chronic health problems, such as high cholesterol, heart disease, arthritis, colds, cancer, and in cases of severe shortage, fatal scurvy.

## What Does Vitamin C Do?

**Neurotransmitters**
*Molecules used as chemical messengers in the body. Serotonin and dopamine are well-known neurotransmitters.*

As we've seen, vitamin C has played an essential role in the development of life on earth. This is apparent when one realizes that vitamin C is utilized by virtually every part of the human body. In fact, there are few, if any, biological functions that do not require vitamin C.

- Vitamin C is a water-soluble antioxidant that protects cells from free radicals. Vitamin C also prevents oxidative damage that leads to the development of atherosclerosis.

- Vitamin C is vital to the immune system, aiding white blood cells that attack and destroy cancer cells, viruses, bacteria, parasites, and other pathogens. Vitamin C also promotes wound healing and acts to control the release of histamine.

- Vitamin C is used by the body to produce collagen, which is used by connective tissues to give strength and shape to our tissues, such as muscles, blood vessels, bones, and teeth.

- Vitamin C helps the body utilize folic acid (required for maintaining DNA) and regulates the uptake of iron (needed for production of hemo-globin, the oxygen-carrying part of blood cells).

- Vitamin C is important for the synthesis of brain neurotransmitters, such as noradrenaline (for energy and mood) and serotonin (for sleep, well-being, and pain control).

## The Many Faces of Vitamin C

As we've seen, the history of human evolution is intimately linked with the development of vitamin C as a vital nutrient that promotes and sustains life on earth. In the following chapters, we'll see how vitamin C pro-motes oxidation—necessary for life-giving energy—while pro-

**Oxidation**
*Refers to the loss of electrons in a chemical reaction. In the body, oxidation is used to "burn" fuel to provide energy for all life processes.*

tecting us from the dangerous byproducts of oxidation, free radicals. And we'll learn how vita-min C helps to form collagen, the basic tissues that hold our bodies together and help shape and strengthen every tissue, from bones and blood vessels to eyes and skin.

Together these and other properties form the underlying basis for the numerous health benefits attributed to vitamin C in more than 10,000 pub-lished scientific papers. To quote from *The Vitamin Connection* by Drs. Cheraskin, Ringsdorf, and Sis-ley, "There is not one body process (such as what goes on inside cells or tissues) and not one disease or syndrome (from the common cold to leprosy) that is not influenced—directly or indirectly—by vitamin C."

# CHAPTER 2

# THE ULTIMATE ANTIOXIDANT

**P**robably the most well known of all of vitamin C's benefits are its powerful antioxidant properties that protect us from the damaging effects of oxidation. Oxidation is the chemical process in which oxygen molecules combine with other molecules to release energy. In addition to producing energy, oxidation produces byproducts. A common, everyday example of an oxygen byproduct is rust, the result of oxygen oxidizing iron. Another example is water, the product of oxygen combining with hydrogen. In the body, cells oxidize sugar (glucose) to produce the energy they need to function.

> **Antioxidants**
> *Substances that contribute a spare electron to neutralize damaging free radicals and render them harmless.*

Even as it produces energy to make life possible, oxidation also has a negative side. When oxygen combines with other molecules, the chemical reaction often results in the production of unstable molecules that contain unpaired electrons. Since electrons are normally paired with other electrons, these unpaired fragments—called free radicals— seek out new electrons in order to return to a state of balance (a landmark discovery by Linus Pauling that led to his first Nobel Prize in 1954).

In the process of stealing electrons, free radicals cause immense damage to tissues, tearing up cell membranes and damaging DNA. Free radicals can also damage the genes in a cell and impair the cell (and any of its descendants) from performing its normal functions. Ironically, this is the very process that may have caused the loss of our gene for making vitamin C in the first place. Additionally, when stealing electrons from other sources, free radicals can set off a chain reaction, or cascade, of continuous reactions that create even more free radicals. These then contribute to even greater damage and set the stage for a number of health problems.

Free-radical damage to cells throughout the body is thought to be a primary factor in the diseases of aging, and maybe of aging itself. The Free Radical Theory of Aging suggests that if we can take steps to minimize this damage, we can slow the aging process. As our knowledge of free-radical chemistry has expanded in the last half of the twentieth century, so too has our appreciation for antioxidants that can prevent or slow the devastating effects of oxidation and the production of free radicals.

## Internal Production of Free Radicals

Free radicals come from several sources. Most are produced in our bodies from normal cellular processes. These endogenous (within the body) free radicals are produced from a number of normal metabolic functions. First, every cell in our bodies produces free radicals as a byproduct of oxidizing (burning) fuel and oxygen to make the energy that is essential for life. This process is a major source of free radicals—each cell in your body produces about 20 billion free radicals every day!

Free radicals are also produced by white blood cells. When the body is under attack, the immune system directs white blood cells, called phagocytes, to release huge amounts of free radicals in a process called phagocytosis. These free radicals act like molecular "bullets" that tear into, and rip apart, invading bacteria, viruses, and parasites. When the body is fighting a chronic infection, this defense mechanism can go out of control and generate massive amounts of free radicals that spill over and damage healthy cells. This problem is associated with a number of degenerative and inflammatory conditions, including arthritis, heart disease, and cancer.

Other causes of rampant free-radical production are burns, surgery, exposure to toxins, infectious and autoimmune diseases, allergies, and severe trauma. All of these conditions promote inflammation, which injures cells, causing further release of even more free radicals.

Free radicals are also produced from normal bodily functions that involve 1) the burning (oxidation) of polyunsaturated fats, 2) the breakdown and elimination of toxic chemicals, drugs, and pesticides, and 3) the increased production of hormones in response to stress.

## External Sources of Free Radicals

When free radicals assault us from external sources, they are referred to as exogenous (outside the body) free radicals. External sources of free radicals include high heat, ultraviolet light, cigarette smoke, air pollution, x-rays, electromagnetic emissions, and other forms of low-level radiation. Exposure to trace metals, such as lead, mercury, iron, and copper, can also promote the production of free radicals.

Free radicals generated from internal and external sources can have a tremendous, and dangerous, impact on human health. In 1954, Dr. Denham Harman proposed that a lifetime of exposure to free radicals is a major cause of aging. Harmon also believed that free radicals contribute to the development of diseases such as heart disease, diabetes, arthritis, and cancer. In his groundbreaking paper, "The Free Radical Theory of Aging," Dr. Harman also proposed that antioxidants, such as vitamin C, could be used to control free radicals, protect DNA, and reduce the incidence of diseases and human aging.

## Antioxidants Quench Free Radicals

Just as the human body bristles with free radicals produced by internal energy production and detoxification processes, it is also equipped with a sophisticated defense system of specialized antioxidants that protect us from free-radical damage. These include lipoic acid and antioxidants enzymes, such as superoxide dismutase (SOD). We also get antioxidants from our diets. Chief among the dietary antioxidants are the vitamins A, $B_6$, C, and E. Other nutrients, such as carotenoids, the amino acids cysteine and taurine, and the mineral selenium, have been proven to provide substantial antioxidant protection when consumed from either foods or supplements.

## Vitamin C—The Ultimate Antioxidant

Remember, early life forms adapted in an environment that was very low in oxygen. As we know, oxygen is an essential ingredient for life, required for energy production and other vital metabolic functions. In order to compete for this scarce resource, early organisms learned to manufacture vitamin C, which then allowed cells to latch on to and capture oxygen molecules. Just as vitamin C aided early life forms by scavenging scarce oxygen from the atmosphere, all life today depends on vitamin C. It acts as a water-soluble antioxidant to control free-radical damage, a byproduct of oxidation.

In the body, vitamin C works in concert with a number of other antioxidants, including vitamin E, lipoic acid, and glutathione. These antioxidants interact in a complex recycling process that resembles an old-fashioned fireman's bucket brigade, where buckets of water are passed, hand over hand, down a line to quench a burning fire. In this case, the body passes a dangerous free radical from one antioxidant to another, reducing its energy (and its potential to damage tissues) with each passing.

The process starts when vitamin E donates an electron to reduce a free radical back to a non-threatening compound. But in doing this, vitamin E turns into a free radical, though one that is far less damaging than the original one. At this point, vitamin C steps in to donate an electron, and vitamin E reverts back to being an antioxidant. The newly regenerated vitamin E molecule goes back to work fighting free radicals, leaving behind another new free radical in the form of an unstable form of vitamin C called dehydroascorbate. Dehydroascorbate is normally regenerated by electron(s) generated by the *mitochondria*, tiny structures in every cell that act as powerhouses to provide energy. The process is repeated until all of the free radicals are eventually quenched. Dehydroascorbate has a half-life in the body of only a few minutes, so if it does not regain its electrons within a few minutes, it is irreversibly lost and eventually passes out of the body in the urine.

**Dehydro-ascorbate**
*Vitamin C that has donated its electrons and is no longer able to act as an antioxidant.*

As we'll see later in this book, large doses, or megadoses, of vitamin C are frequently used to treat very serious diseases, infections, and cancer. In such large doses, vitamin C is not used for any of its proven metabolic or biochemical actions. Megadoses of vitamin C are employed strictly as a "delivery vehicle" to donate electrons to be used in the battle against the free radicals that are generated by disease processes. When used in this manner, vitamin C is "sacrificed" for its electrons, and then eliminated by the body as dehydroascorbate.

# CHAPTER 3

# VITAMIN C SUPPORTS HEALTHY SKIN, JOINTS, AND VISION

One of vitamin C's most vital roles in human health is in the production and maintenance of collagen. Collagen is a protein that makes up the connective tissues found throughout the body, especially in the skin, ligaments, cartilage, bones, and teeth. The most abundant protein in the body, it accounts for more mass than all the other proteins put together.

Collagen acts as a kind of intracellular "glue" that gives support, shape, and bulk to blood vessels, bones, and organs such as the heart, kidneys, and liver. Collagen fibers keep bones and blood vessels strong, and help to anchor our teeth to our gums. Collagen is also required for the repair of blood vessels, bruises, and broken bones.

Vitamin C is essential for the formation of collagen. While many vitamins and minerals act as catalysts to support the manufacture of proteins, in the case of collagen, vitamin C is actually used up as it combines with amino acids, such as lysine, glycine, and proline, to form procollagen. Procollagen is then used to manufacture one of several types of collagen that can be used for different tissues throughout the body. There are at least fourteen different types of collagen in the body, but the most common ones are:

**Type I.** Makes up the fibers found in connective

tissues of the skin, bone, teeth, tendons, and ligaments.

**Type II.** Round fibers found in cartilage.

**Type III.** Forms connective tissues that give shape and strength to organs, such as the liver, heart, and kidneys.

**Type IV.** Forms sheets that lie between layers of cells in the blood vessels, muscles, and eyes.

## Vitamin C Deficiency Equals Collagen Deficiency

Our bodies are continually manufacturing collagen to maintain and repair connective tissues lost to daily wear and tear. Without vitamin C, collagen formation is disrupted, resulting in a wide variety of problems throughout the body. Scurvy, the disease caused by vitamin C deficiency, is really a process that disrupts the body's ability to manufacture collagen and connective tissues. When a person is suffering from scurvy, his or her body literally falls apart as collagen is broken down and not replaced. The joints begin to wear down as tendons shrivel and weaken. The blood vessels crumble and begin to fall apart, leading to bruising and bleeding as vessels rupture (hemorrhage) throughout the body. Teeth loosen and fall out as the gums and the connective tissues holding teeth also begin to erode. Organs, once held firmly together by connective tissues, also lose structural strength and begin to fail. In time, the various body tissues weaken, and the immune system and heart give out, leading to death.

## Arthritis

Arthritis is a localized degeneration of joint cartilage, mainly affecting the weight-bearing joints.

More common in the elderly and in those who are overweight, arthritis is also caused by the mechanical stresses and major trauma that result from sports injuries. Arthritis causes aching in the joints, limitation of movement and range of motion, and a loss of dexterity. A "wear-and-tear disease of aging," arthritis generally begins in middle age, and by age sixty, most people have some degree of osteoarthritis.

Arthritis is caused by a breakdown in cellular processes that produce, maintain, and repair cartilage. Physical stress on joints causes destruction of collagen and may also inhibit its production. When the body is unable to make enough collagen, or when there is an excessive amount of destruction of the collagen matrix, the joints start to erode.

## Conventional Treatment for Arthritis

Modern medicine utilizes several classes of drugs to treat arthritis, including analgesics, corticosteroids, uric acid–lowering drugs, immunosuppressive drugs, nonsteroidal anti-inflammatory drugs (NSAIDs), and disease-modifying anti-rheumatic drugs (DMARDs), such as antimalarial drugs, gold compounds, penicillamine, and sulfasalazine.

While many of these drugs provide temporary relief of pain and inflammation, they have little or no effect on the underlying disease processes. In fact, many drugs, such as the NSAIDs, actually worsen the condition by suppressing the normal tissue-building processes. Additionally, long-term toxicity and side effects associated with many approved arthritis drugs frequently require that patients be carefully monitored and reevaluated by their physicians.

## Nutritional Approaches for Arthritis

Alternative nutritional approaches for arthritis have

become popular over the last decade. The most popular supplements include joint-building substances, such as chondroitin sulfate, glucosamine, and SAMe (S-adenosyl methionine). Other supplements include anti-inflammatory substances, such as *Boswellia serrata*, turmeric, and essential fatty acids (EFAs).

## Vitamin C for Arthritis

As we have seen, one of vitamin C's most vital functions is the production and maintenance of collagen, the tough protein that makes up the connective tissues found in our joints. The type I collagen that lines our joints is composed of a combination of vitamin C and amino acids, such as lycine, glycine, and proline. When vitamin C levels are low or become depleted, our ability to produce collagen may not be able to keep up with the constant loss of connective tissues lining our joints.

Research has shown that vitamin C can aid in reducing the pain, inflammation, and swelling of arthritis. Vitamin C can also support healthy joint functions and keep joints, particularly the knees, flexible and comfortable. Recent studies have found that vitamin C can help to reduce the progression of arthritis. After looking at the records of 640 individuals enrolled in a large study, researchers found that people taking 420 mg of vitamin C per day had a 300 percent reduction in the progression of their arthritis compared with those taking only minimal RDA levels.

This favorable effect of vitamin C was found to be due to a reduction in the loss of joint cartilage. This effect was believed to be due to vitamin C's role in making new cartilage. An additional benefit seen with higher doses of vitamin C was a significant reduction in knee pain.

In addition to the joint degeneration and loss of

connective tissue that are seen in osteoarthritis, rheumatoid arthritis also involves alterations in the inflammatory response of the body. One characteristic of rheumatoid arthritis is excessive immune-system activity caused by the body's efforts to clear out the cellular debris being shed by degrading joint tissues. This results in a huge amount of free-radical activity within the joint and leads to further inflammation of the tissues. Researchers have recently found that blood levels of vitamin C are extremely low in people with rheumatoid arthritis. This suggests that vitamin C may also protect against further damage to inflamed joints.

## Vitamin C Reduces Risk of Cataracts

A recent study suggests that vitamin C can help to reduce the formation of cataracts. In a study published in the *American Journal of Clinical Nutrition,* researchers investigated the link between vitamin C and the incidence of age-related cataracts. At the beginning of the study, the researchers enrolled 492 women, aged fifty-three to seventy-three, who were free of cataracts. They then carefully measured how much vitamin C the women consumed over the next fifteen years.

For women younger than sixty years old, vitamin C consumption greater than 362 mg per day was found to reduce the risk of developing cataracts by 57 percent when compared with women who took less than 140 mg per day. And women who used vitamin C supplements for at least ten years reduced their risk of developing cataracts by 60 percent when compared with women who didn't consume any supplemental vitamin C.

**Cataract**
*A clouding of the normally transparent crystalline lens of the eye that disrupts the ability to clearly focus images on the retina.*

Beauty is in the eye of the beholder, and so is the knowledge that something as simple as four or five daily servings of orange juice (or a vitamin C capsule) will help people preserve vision far into the golden years.

# CHAPTER 4

# VITAMIN C PROTECTS AGAINST HEART DISEASE AND STROKE

In this chapter, we will see how vitamin C saves lives, prevents atherosclerosis, aids in the removal of cholesterol deposits from arterial walls, and regulates high blood pressure. A recent large study found that men who take vitamin C supplements live, on average, six years longer than men who get their vitamin C only from dietary sources. This very significant increase in life span seems to be due to a sharp reduction in deaths from heart disease. Based on this study, it has been estimated that if everyone took several hundred milligrams of vitamin C a day, more than 100,000 lives and $100 billion in healthcare costs would be saved each year in just the United States alone.

## Cardiovascular Disease and Stroke

Cardiovascular disease, especially heart attacks and strokes, kill at least 12 million people across the globe each year. And in the United States, heart attacks and strokes remain the primary cause of mortality, accounting for a full 50 percent of all deaths.

Strokes occur when a blood clot (thrombosis) blocks a blood vessel or artery (cerebral infarction), or when a blood vessel breaks, interrupting blood flow to an area of the brain (hemorrhagic stroke). These processes cause the immediate death of brain cells in the affected area. Additionally, as brain cells die, they rupture and release a number of dangerous chemicals in a chain reaction called the "ischemic cascade." These chemicals then spread out and cause even more damage to the *penumbra,* which means "the cells surrounding the area."

Research published in the medical journal *Stroke* reports that people with high blood levels of vitamin C have a significantly lower risk of having a stroke. The findings were based on measurements of vitamin C blood levels in more than 2,120 men and women living in rural Japan. From 1977 to 1997, researchers logged a total of 196 strokes in the volunteers. After comparing vitamin C levels, the scientists discovered that people with the lowest levels of vitamin C faced a 70 percent increased risk of stroke than those with the highest levels of vitamin C in their blood. Of the 196 strokes, 109 were caused by a blockage of blood flow (infarction), 54 were caused by hemorrhagic stroke, and 33 were of undetermined types. The researchers commented on the importance of the study, stating, "This is the first prospective study to make the correlation between vitamin C in the bloodstream and incidence of stroke."

**Stroke**
*The third leading cause of death in the U.S. It occurs when a region of the brain loses blood flow, usually from an obstructed blood vessel. Each year about 400,000 cases of stroke and approximately 150,000 deaths from it are reported in the U.S.*

Because both types of stroke were reduced, researchers speculated that the protective effect of vitamin C went well beyond its well-known antioxidant actions. Cerebral infarctions are caused by atherosclerosis (blocked arteries), which can be prevented by the antioxidant effects of vitamin C. Hemorrhagic strokes, on the other hand, result from ruptured blood vessels. Therefore, the proven role of vitamin C in building collagen and strengthening connective tissues in the blood vessels seems to explain this significant reduction in hemorrhagic strokes.

## Atherosclerosis

Atherosclerosis, or "hardening of the arteries," is a primary cause of heart disease. It often starts early in life as a mass of sticky fatty compounds that gradually builds up on the inner lining of arteries to form a thick "plaque." This process usually develops over a period of years or decades, until deposits become so thick that they begin to block the coronary arteries and restrict blood flow. Atherosclerosis can suddenly appear as chest pains (angina), but sometimes the first (and last) warning is a sudden—and often, fatal—heart attack. Early symptoms of atherosclerosis can include:

1. Chest pains with physical exertion (angina) caused by a blockage of the coronary arteries. If an artery is completely blocked, the result can be a heart attack.

2. Memory loss or temporary disorientation or sensory loss (transient ischemic attacks, temporary "mini-strokes") can be a sign of a blockage of arteries leading to the brain. Complete blockage often results in a stroke.

3. Pain felt in the calves after walking relatively short distances (intermittent claudication) is a sign of a blockage of the arteries in the leg.

All of these symptoms are serious signs of significant arterial narrowing in the affected areas, as well as elsewhere in the body.

## Risk Factors for Atherosclerosis

Some of the many risk factors known to increase

the likelihood of developing atherosclerosis and heart disease include:

- Smoking.

- Hypertension (high blood pressure).

- Diabetes.

- Elevated cholesterol.

- Sedentary lifestyle.

- Obesity.

- Family history of heart disease.

- Stress.

## Medical Treatment of Atherosclerosis

Over the last two decades, nutritionist and doctors have recommended various lifestyle modifications to reduce atherosclerosis. These include quitting smoking, losing weight, cutting back on dietary intake of cholesterol and fatty foods, and regular, moderate exercise. In some cases, doctors will prescribe drugs, such as ACE inhibitors, beta-blockers, and lipid-lowering statin drugs. Yet, even when following all the current guidelines and therapies, many people will still develop coronary artery disease, carotid artery disease, or other vascular illness.

**Atherosclerosis**
*A disease characterized by narrow arteries caused by cholesterol-rich plaque. Risk factors include elevated cholesterol and triglyceride levels, high blood pressure, and cigarette smoking.*

When traditional therapies fail, surgery is often the last resort. Surgeons operate to replace, or "bypass," blocked arteries by grafting veins harvested from the legs in an attempt to restore blood flow to the heart. Alternately, balloon angioplasty attempts to restore blood flow in constricted arteries by literally smashing the plaque against the arterial walls to increase the diameter of the arteries. As impressive as these surgical advances are, they also present a number of serious side effects, including death, and even when successful, the results are often temporary and blockages can reappear within months.

## Vitamin C Improves Blood Flow

The ability of blood vessels to relax and open up to blood flow (dilate) is severely reduced in people with atherosclerosis. Much of the damage to the heart during a heart attack, and to the brain during a stroke, is caused by the inability of blood vessels to open enough to allow blood to flow to the affected areas. The chest pains of angina are also caused by the inability of the coronary arteries to dilate. Doses of as little as 500 mg of vitamin C per day have consistently been proven to improve dilation of blood vessels in people with atherosclerosis, angina pectoris, congestive heart failure, and high blood pressure.

## Vitamin C Lowers Cholesterol

Scientists have known for decades that dangerously high levels of cholesterol, known as hypercholesterolemia, are accompanied by very low blood levels of vitamin C. In 1981, researchers discovered that vitamin C plays a vital role in reducing cholesterol levels, by enhancing the conversion of cholesterol to bile salts that can be easily eliminated by the body. This has been supported by several large studies that proved that vitamin C can reduce the incidence of cardiovascular diseases, lower cholesterol levels, and increase the ratio of the so-called "good" cholesterol, high-density lipoprotein (HDL). When researchers gave volunteers 1 gram of vitamin C per day for three months, cholesterol levels declined by 10 percent and triglyceride levels dropped by 40 percent. A second study also found that 3 g of vitamin C every day dropped cholesterol levels an impressive 18 percent, and triglycerides by 12 percent in only three weeks.

**Triglycerides**
*Molecules formed when three fatty acids are linked together by a single molecule of a type of alcohol called glycerol.*

In 1994, researchers from the USDA and National Institute on Aging conducted a trial on participants in the Baltimore Longitudinal Study of Aging to investigate the effect of vitamin C on total cholesterol levels. The researchers found that vitamin C intake that greatly exceeded the RDA of 60 mg per day resulted in a significant rise in levels of the desirable form of HDL cholesterol. The researchers stated that, in order to see positive changes in cholesterol profiles, people had to increase their intake of vitamin C to between four and five times the recommended daily dose (between 215 and 345 mg per day).

## Linus Pauling Challenges Cholesterol Theories

In 1989, the eminent American scientist and two-time Nobel Prize winner Linus Pauling announced a breakthrough in how we view and treat heart disease. In "A Unified Theory of Human Cardiovascular Disease," Linus Pauling announced that the deposits of plaque seen in atherosclerosis were not the *cause* of heart disease, but were actually the *result* of our bodies trying to repair the damage caused by long-term vitamin C deficiency. In essence, Pauling believed that heart disease is a form of scurvy, and plaque is the body's attempt to reinforce and patch weakened blood vessels and arteries that would otherwise rupture. Pauling also showed that heart disease can be easily prevented or treated by taking vitamin C and other supplements.

## Plaque Deposits

Pauling based his revolutionary theory on a number of important scientific findings. First was the discovery that plaque deposits found in human aortas are made up of a special form of cholesterol called lipoprotein (a) or Lp(a), not from ordinary LDL cholesterol, as mainstream science had once believed. Lp(a) is a special form of LDL cholesterol that we now know binds to form the thick sheets of plaque that obstruct arteries.

Another finding central to Pauling's theory was the observation that plaque deposits are not formed randomly throughout the circulatory system. This was first reported in the early 1950s when a Canadian doctor, G. C. Willis, M.D., observed that plaque always forms nearest the heart, where blood vessels and arteries are constantly being stretched and bent, rather than being spread evenly throughout the entire cardiovascular system. Willis also noted that damage to vessels that triggers plaque deposits always occurs in regions that are exposed to the highest blood pressures, such as the aorta, where blood is forcefully ejected from the heart.

**Aorta**
*The largest artery in the body. It carries blood from the heart through the chest and into the abdomen where it divides and goes to each leg.*

In 1985, a team of researchers verified that plaque forms only in areas of the artery that become damaged. Just as cracks form in a garden hose that has become weak and worn from constant bending and high pressure, cracks form in the lining of the arterial wall. As these tiny cracks open up, they expose strands of the amino acid lysine (one of the primary components of collagen) to the bloodstream. It is these strands that initially attract Lp(a). Lp(a) is an especially "sticky form of cholesterol that is attracted to lysine. Drawn to the break, Lp(a) begins to collect and attach to the exposed strands. As Lp(a) covers the lysine strands, free lysine in the blood is drawn to the growing deposit. This process continues as lysine and Lp(a) are both drawn from the blood to build ever-larger deposits of plaque. Over time, this process gradually reduces the inner diameter of the vessels and restricts its capacity to carry the blood.

## Heart Disease as Low-Level Scurvy

Observing the newly described process of plaque formation, Pauling recognized a similarity to the underlying processes seen in scurvy. He also saw similarities between human and animal models of atherosclerosis that pointed to a connection with scurvy. First, cardiovascular disease does not occur in any of the animals that are able to manufacture their own vitamin C. As pointed out earlier, many animals produce large amounts of vitamin C that are equivalent to human doses ranging from 10–20 g per day. Second, the *only* animals that produce Lp(a) are those who, like humans, have also lost the ability to produce their own vitamin C.

Putting all the pieces of the puzzle together, Pauling recognized that the ability to form plaque is really the body's attempt to repair damage caused by a long-term deficiency of vitamin C. He knew that early in humanity's evolution, our ancestors lived in tropical regions where the diet consisted primarily of fruits and vegetables. With a daily intake estimated to be in the range of several hundred milligrams to several grams per day, our ancestors easily survived the loss of the gene required to manufacture vitamin C. Almost unnoticed, this mutation was passed on to successive generations, and only became a problem when early humans began to spread to other regions of the world. In effect, when humankind left the "garden," the lack of a reliable and adequate supply of dietary vitamin C led to scurvy.

Pauling thought that scurvy was one of the greatest threats to humankind's early survival, and believed that the loss of blood during times of vitamin C deficiency, particularly during the ice ages, likely brought humans close to the point of extinction.

## Plaque as a Lifesaver

Evolution works by a process of trial and error that, over the course of millions of years, favors the selection of traits that increase the survival of a species. The core of Pauling's theory is that, over time, evolutionary pressures forced the body to develop a repair mechanism that would allow it to cope with the damage caused by chronic vitamin C deficiency. The repair mechanism is as elegant as it is simple. When arteries became weak and began to rupture, the body responded by "gluing" the damaged areas together with Lp(a) to prevent a slow death from internal bleeding. In essence, plaque is the body's attempt to patch blood vessels damaged by low-level scurvy. Accordingly, Pauling believed that conventional "triggers" of plaque formation, such as homocysteine and oxidized cholesterol, are actually just additional symptoms of scurvy.

## Scientific Support for Pauling's Unified Theory

Pauling's theory was unique in that it addressed a fact never explained by older, mainstream theories. Specifically, Pauling finally explained why plaque isn't randomly distributed throughout the body, but restricted to areas of high mechanical stress. A surprising number of animal studies have been found to support Pauling's theory. Research conducted with animals that cannot make their own vitamin C found that when vitamin C levels are reduced, collagen production drops and blood vessels become thinner and weaker. Additional studies also confirm that when animals are deprived of vitamin C, their bodies respond by increasing blood levels of Lp(a) and forming plaque deposits to strengthen arteries and prevent vessel ruptures.

## Collagen Melts Plaque, Keeps Arteries Open

In addition to taking vitamin C to prevent atherosclerosis, Pauling recommended a combination of vitamin C and the amino acids lysine and proline to help remove existing plaque while strengthening weak and damaged arteries. Since the body produces collagen from lysine and proline, Pauline reasoned that by increasing concentrations of lysine and proline in the blood, Lp(a) molecules would bind with the free lysine, rather than with the lysine strands exposed by the cracks in blood vessels.

## How Much Vitamin C Prevents Atherosclerosis?

While acute scurvy can be prevented by a mere 10 mg of vitamin C per day, there is no current research showing how much vitamin C might be required to prevent the atherosclerotic plaques of chronic scurvy. In his Unified Theory, Linus Pauling often recommended 3,000 mg per day as an effective dose. Anecdotal reports from patients using the Pauling Therapy indicate that rapid recovery is frequently the rule, not the exception, allowing many people to avoid open heart surgery and angioplasty.

# Vitamin C and High Blood Pressure

Blood pressure is defined as the pressure exerted by the blood against the walls of the blood vessels, especially the arteries. It varies with the strength of the heartbeat, the elasticity of the arterial walls, the volume and viscosity of the blood, and a person's health, age, and physical condition. A normal level is 120/80 where the first number is the systolic pressure and the second is the diastolic pressure.

High blood pressure, or hypertension, is serious health problem and a major risk factor for heart disease and strokes. An estimated 25 percent of Americans suffer from the effects of hypertension. Hypertension is associated with atherosclerosis, hypertensive renal failure, stroke, congestive heart failure, and "myocardial infarction," or heart attacks. Although hypertension has been extensively studied, more than 90 percent of all cases are referred to as "essential hypertension," meaning the cause of the elevated blood pressure is unknown. Regardless of the cause, a large body of research from population studies has established that vitamin C can significantly reduce the high blood pressure of hypertensive patients.

In a recent study conducted by researchers at the Boston University School of Medicine and the Linus Pauling Institute at Oregon State University, forty-five patients were given either 500 mg of vitamin C or a placebo, daily. At the beginning of the study, average systolic pressure was 155, and diastolic pressure was 87. After a month, there was no significant change in those receiving the placebo, while those taking vitamin C had a drop in total blood pressure measurements

**Placebo**

*A "sugar pill" or other inactive substance often used in studies to help researchers determine the effects of a drug or other active substance being tested*

of 9 percent. Specifically, average systolic readings dropped from 155 to 142, and diastolic readings dropped from 87 to 79. Significantly, the research showed that taking vitamin C had no effect on people with normal blood pressure levels.

## Vitamin C Relaxes Blood Vessels

In a series of related studies, scientists have shown that 500 mg of vitamin C daily can improve blood pressure by allowing blood vessels to relax. The research also shows that by increasing the endothelial function of blood vessels, vitamin C can help to control or prevent angina (chest pains) and reduce the risk of a heart attack or stroke.

**Endothelial**
*Refers to the cells that line and protect the inside portion of the arteries and vessels that are exposed to the bloodstream.*

The researchers speculate that vitamin C helps to control blood pressure by acting as an antioxidant to help protect the body's level of nitric oxide (NO). Nitric oxide is a natural compound that is manufactured in the body to act as a neurotransmitter, or "messenger molecule." In the cardiovascular system, nitric oxide acts by relaxing blood vessels to help the body maintain normal, healthy blood pressure.

When antioxidant levels are low, or when we encounter chronic stress in our lives, oxidative stresses can inhibit, and actually inactivate, nitric oxide in our bodies, leading to high blood pressure. Vitamin C helps to protect nitric oxide so it can perform its normal function of regulating blood pressure. Additionally, vitamin C is far safer, not to mention less expensive, than the prescription drugs currently used to reduce high blood pressure.

CHAPTER 5

# VITAMIN C FIGHTS COLDS AND PROVIDES IMMUNE SUPPORT

Vitamin C is required for the proper functioning of the immune system. Following the publication of Linus Pauling's book *Vitamin C and the Common Cold* in 1970, use of large doses of vitamin C (greater than 1 gram per day) to prevent colds and other infections increased dramatically. Vitamin C is required for the production of the white blood cells, T cells, and macrophages that defend us against viruses, bacteria, parasites, and cancer.

Vitamin C also increases the production of antibodies, boosts production of interferon, and helps to coordinate the cellular immune response. In short, vitamin C supports the immune system as it responds to constant threats from bacterial, viral, and fungal diseases. When vitamin C levels are low or become depleted, the body cannot mount an effective response to defend our health.

## Vitamin C and the Common Cold

Large doses of vitamin C (2 g or more per day) can dramatically shorten both the duration and severity of a cold if taken at first sign of symptoms. Most studies show that vitamin C therapy can result in milder symptoms while reducing the duration by about a third.

More than twenty studies have found that taking vitamin C preventively reduces the annual number of colds in children. One study of more than 600 children, between the ages of eight and nine, found that 1,000 mg of vitamin C a day for three months reduced the severity and duration of colds, but not the number of colds. To understand how vitamin C can help us recover from colds, flu, and other forms of infection, we need to understand that vitamin C takes on a new role when the body is under attack.

## Common Cold as "Acute Induced Scurvy"

Often, we may begin to notice that we are starting to feel ill, only to have the symptoms quickly disappear within a day or so. This is what is supposed to happen when the immune system is healthy and well supported. At the first sign of an attack, all of the components of the immune complex move quickly to identify, target, and kill the invading pathogens.

**Immune System**
*A complex system of responses that fight invaders such as bacteria and viruses.*

Just as often, we don't get better and our symptoms worsen as we are caught up in a cold or flu that can last for days or weeks. The invading viruses have slipped past our first lines of defense, damaging the energy-producing mitochondria in our cells. This damage results in a flood of free radicals that quickly use up all the vitamin C in the affected area, such as the nose and throat. Dr. Robert Cathcart, a pioneer in the field of orthomolecular medicine, refers to this condition as "acute induced scurvy."

When vitamin C is depleted in the affected area, the body can no longer mount an effective response until it has produced enough antibodies to attack and destroy the virus. In the meantime, the condition has time to spread to the sinuses, to the ears, and even to the lungs. This also allows bacteria to take advantage of the situation, potentially causing secondary infections, such as bronchitis, pneumonia, or worse.

Cathcart believes that taking moderate doses of vitamin C (that is, 200–2,000 mg per day) in such conditions may prevent the spread of the infection to other area of the body, but will do little to shorten the course of the illness. On the other hand, Cathcart argues that taking megadoses of vitamin C can force enough electrons into the affected tissues to neutralize all the free radicals and support the white cells that "come out fighting mad and destroy all the viruses." "It does not matter that the disease is moderately advanced," states Cathcart, if sufficient C is used, "the cold will be shortly terminated."

> **Orthomolecular**
> *Refers to the eradication of disease by giving the body the "right molecules" it needs to stay healthy.*

## The Power of Megadose Vitamin C

Building on the groundbreaking work of Linus Pauling, Irwin Stone, and other orthomolecular physicians, Cathcart has helped to shape our understanding of megadose vitamin therapy, which uses vitamin C in doses higher than those required for normal cellular functions. When taken in very high doses (10–100 g or more per day, depending upon the person and the illness), vitamin C works in a uniquely different way to fight off serious illness.

We've seen that vitamin C is required to help protect the body from the ravages of free radicals and for the constant repair of our connective tissues. And, except for losses due to collagen formation, most of the time vitamin C is recycled by the body's antioxidant system. But when the body is challenged by cancer, colds, or other diseases, vitamin C takes on a new role. Dr. Cathcart and other proponents of megadose therapy contend that when we become seriously ill, the body is overwhelmed by a flood of free radicals that quickly use up all of the available stores of vitamin C. This impairs the immune response, which depends on vitamin C to mount an effective defense against the invading organisms (or tumor, in the case of cancer).

By ingesting or infusing large amounts of vitamin C, the aim is to saturate the body with enough electrons to destroy all of the free radicals being generated in the tissues affected by the disease. In short, the body is using the electrons donated by vitamin C, and then tossing away the dehydro-ascorbate.

## The Controversy Surrounding Megadose Therapy

Megadose vitamin C therapy continues to be a highly controversial topic. Traditional medicine tends to view vitamin C as a nutrient that is useful only for preventing scurvy. In "The Third Face of Vitamin C," published in *The Journal of Orthomolecular Medicine* in 1993, Dr. Cathcart detailed his clinical experience treating more than 20,000 patients with high doses of vitamin C over a twenty-three-year period. Cathcart found that doses of up to 200 or more grams per day were effective in treating all diseases involving free radicals. These include infections, cardiovascular diseases, cancer, trauma, burns (both thermal and radiation), surgeries, allergies, autoimmune diseases, and aging.

Megadose therapy has caught the interest and fired the imagination of many eminent researchers. The late Irwin Stone pioneered the early use of high dose vitamin C in the treatment of disease. His close friend Dr. Frederick Klenner conducted much of the original clinical research on vitamin C megadose therapy, reporting that most viral diseases could be cured when patients were treated with intravenous sodium ascorbate in amounts up to 200 g per day.

**Intravenous (IV)**
*Refers to the administration of a drug or nutrient with a steel needle or plastic catheter inserted into a vein.*

Klenner is credited with bringing megadose therapy to the attention of Linus Pauling. Pauling went on to conduct research with the Scottish surgeon Ewan Cameron showing that high-dose vitamin C therapy doubled the life span of cancer patients. (See "Vitamin C Extends the Life Spans of People with Cancer" on page 51.)

Based on their work, a large number of physicians now routinely use massive doses of vitamin C in their clinical practice for the treatment of a wide variety of diseases. Nevertheless, most physicians still remain critical of these treatments, convinced that the usefulness of vitamin C is limited to the prevention of scurvy.

# CHAPTER 6

# VITAMIN C
# AND CANCER

In the 1940s, scientists and medical researchers began to notice a strong connection between low blood levels of vitamin C and an increase in the incidence of several forms of cancer. Studies conducted over the last several decades have confirmed this link, consistently showing that eating a diet of fresh fruits and vegetables high in vitamin C can result in a significant reduction of many types of cancer. This profound anticancer benefit forms the basis for dietary guidelines issued by the National Cancer Institute recommending the consumption of at least five servings of fruits and vegetables per day. In addition to vitamin C, fruits and vegetables are also a significant source of fiber and a variety of vitamins and minerals.

## Vitamin C Prevents Cancer

Vitamin C helps the body prevent cancer in a number of ways. First, research shows that vitamin C exerts anticancer effects by acting as a powerful antioxidant to prevent the oxidation of fats that can form powerful cancer-promoting compounds. When scientists gave elderly patients 400 mg of vitamin C per day for as little as one year, they noted a significant reduction in the blood serum levels of these dangerous compounds.

Second, vitamin C works inside of our cells to reduce the effects of free radicals. Free radicals attack cellular targets, such as cell membranes, proteins, and nucleic acids, and cause structural damage to DNA. These genetic alterations appear as mutations and chromosomal alterations in certain genes that are known to cause various forms of cancer and increase the risk of developing cancer later in life.

**Carcinogen**
*Chemical substance or mixtures of chemical substances that are known to induce cancer or increase its incidence.*

Third, vitamin C aids the body's detoxifying systems by stimulating the production of liver enzymes that break down and eliminate dangerous environmental pollutants and toxins that are known to have powerful mutagenic or carcinogenic effects.

Additionally, vitamin C reduces the risk of developing cancer by preventing the formation of cancer-causing chemicals called nitrosamines. These are formed when bacteria in the stomach metabolize nitrate, a nitrogen compound found in fish and leafy green and root vegetables, such as spinach and carrots. Nitrosamines are also added to processed and cured meats, such as ham, bacon, and sausages, to prevent bacterial growth.

Researchers believe that the relatively high consumption of orange juice by people living in citrus-producing regions of the United States may explain the lower number of reported cases of cancers of the large bowel in those areas. Researchers have found that vitamin C significantly reduces urinary levels of nitrosamines in humans. Animal studies also show that vitamin C protects against nitrosamine-induced cancer by inhibiting and reducing the formation of tumors in treated animals.

## Vitamin C Fights Tumor Growth

Even as cancer cells begin to spread, vitamin C

plays an important role in fighting tumor growth. Dr. Ewan Cameron theorized that as cancer cells grow, they must first invade other cells to open up space for tumor expansion. In order to invade these adjoining cells, tumors must first break through the tough cell walls that are held together with "intercellular cement," as Pauling referred to the connective tissues and chains of collagen that hold cells together.

In order to break down these connective tissues and invade the tissues, cancer cells release an enzyme called hyaluronidase that weakens and breaks down connective tissues. Cancer cells also produce a second enzyme, called collagenase, which works to dissolve collagen. Under the fierce attack of these two powerful enzymes, cell walls eventually dissolve and collapse, allowing cancer cells to move in and expand.

Vitamin C is required for the maintenance of the collagen and fibrous materials that make up healthy cells. When vitamin C levels are too low to adequately maintain strong cellular walls, the damage caused by cancer enzymes is allowed to proceed unchecked. In addition to helping slow the progression of cell invasion, vitamin C has also been found to produce a substance that inhibits hyaluronidase. The more vitamin C in the system, the more this inhibitor is released.

## New Mechanism of Action

A letter published in the January 12, 2002 issue of the British medical journal *The Lancet* revealed a new mechanism that helps to explain why vitamin C is helpful in protecting the body against cancer. In their paper, the researchers report that vitamin C inhibits the cancer-causing effects of hydrogen peroxide. Cells must communicate with one another to stay healthy and to promote normal cell

**Hydrogen Peroxide (H$_2$O$_2$)**
*A known tumor promoter that is produced when the body breaks down amino acids and fats for cellular energy.*

growth. Hydrogen peroxide is a known tumor promoter that works, in part, by inhibiting the normal processes of cell-to-cell communication. What the researchers discovered from animal studies is that vitamin C works to inhibit this tumor-promoting property of hydrogen peroxide.

## Studies Show Vitamin C Reduces Incidence of Cancer

In a comprehensive review of studies on vitamin C's protective effects against various types of cancer, the *American Journal of Clinical Nutrition* reported that thirty-three studies showed a significant link between vitamin C intake (defined as 160 mg or more per day) and a lower incidence of cancer. Ongoing research continues to find a protective—as opposed to curative—effect for a number of cancers.

The most significant finding came from a published study involving 11,348 adults over a ten-year period. This study showed that males taking the highest amount of vitamin C had a 45 percent reduction in all causes of mortality, a 22 percent reduction in cancer incidence, and a 42 percent reduction in heart attacks.

### Breast Cancer

Two recent studies have found that higher intake of vitamin C can protect against breast cancer in certain groups of women. The Nurses' Health Study—one of the largest investigations into the risk factors for major chronic diseases in women—found that premenopausal women with a family history of breast cancer who consumed an average of 205 mg of vitamin C per day were 63 percent less likely to develop breast cancer than similar women who consumed only 70 mg of vitamin C per day.

Another study, the Swedish Mammography Cohort, found that overweight women who consumed an average of 110 mg of vitamin C per day had a 39 percent lower risk of breast cancer when compared with overweight women who consumed only 30 mg (or less than half the RDA) of vitamin C per day.

Researchers have also shown that the spread of breast cancer, or metastasis, may be reduced by taking large amounts of vitamin C.

## Mouth, Larynx, and Esophageal Cancer

In Asia, cancer of the mouth, larynx, and esophagus is the leading form of cancer in men, and the third most frequent form of cancer in women. Approximately 30,000 new cases of oral cancer are diagnosed in the United States each year, and about 9,000 people die from oral cancer each year. Research shows that a low intake of vitamin C index is associated with a significantly greater number of cancers of the mouth, larynx, and esophagus.

## Lung Cancer

Researchers reviewed the intake of a group of 870 men over a period of twenty-five years. They found that men who consumed 83 mg or more of vitamin C per day were 64 percent less likely to develop lung cancer, compared with men who consumed less than 63 mg of vitamin C per day.

## Pancreatic Cancer

In one study, high intake of vitamin C was shown to cut the risk of developing pancreatic cancer in half. Other studies also show that eating fruits and vegetables high in vitamin C offers significant protection against pancreatic cancer, which is the fifth leading cause of cancer deaths.

## Digestive-Tract Cancers

A number of studies have proven that increased intake of dietary vitamin C reduces stomach cancer. Scientists believe that vitamin C protects the stomach by inhibiting the formation of carcinogenic compounds in the stomach, such as nitrosamines. Additionally, people infected with the common bacteria *Helicobacter pylori* (*H. pylori*) have a much higher incidence of stomach cancer. Studies have shown that supplemental vitamin C—in addition to standard *H. pylori* eradication therapies—may be effective in reducing the risk of stomach cancer.

Vitamin C–rich foods have been shown to have a significant effect in reducing both colon and rectal cancer. Supplementation with 3 g of vitamin C per day has been found to effectively prevent further polyp growth in colon cancer, and intake of more than 157 mg of vitamin C per day has been found to reduce the risk of developing colon cancer by 50 percent.

## Prostate and Bladder Cancers

In an study presented at the American Institute for Cancer Research 10th Annual Research Conference in September 2001, researchers revealed that vitamin C showed potent activity against two forms of prostate cancer cells, and seven other forms of urinary tract cancers. While vitamin C didn't kill the cancer cells outright, it was found to trigger the breakdown of the malignant DNA in the cells, as well as blocking the growth of the tumors.

Research has also shown that people taking 500 mg of vitamin C per day for ten years or more cut their risk of developing bladder cancer by 60 percent.

## Skin Cancer

Applying vitamin C to the skin can inhibit tumor promotion in mouse skin, according to a recent study. Moreover, ascorbyl palmitate, the fat-soluble form of vitamin C, was found to be at least thirty times more effective than water-soluble vitamin C in tumor reduction. Vitamin C has also been found to reduce the number of malignant skin lesions in mice exposed to high levels of ultraviolet light (UV). Researchers have found similar results in human studies, showing that vitamin C inhibits the formation of cancer-causing compounds in skin exposed to UV radiation.

## Vitamin C Extends the Life Spans of People with Cancer

While a growing number of studies show that a higher intake of vitamin C is associated with significant reductions in many forms of cancer, in general most findings support a preventative, rather than curative, role for vitamin C and cancer.

In 1976, Dr. Linus Pauling reported on the results of cancer research he conducted in collaboration with Ewan Cameron. Pauling and Cameron treated 100 terminally ill cancer patients at the Vale of Leven Hospital in Scotland with very large doses of vitamin C (10 g per day intravenously for ten days followed by at least 10 g per day orally indefinitely). The results of their trial showed that vitamin C therapy was effective in increasing both the survival time and the quality of life of terminal cancer patients. Patients receiving vitamin C lived more than four times longer than 1,000 control subjects who received no vitamin C. Only 3 of these 1,000 patients survived for more than a year, while 16 of the 100 patients taking vitamin C lived a year or longer.

More recently, Cameron has reported similar results from a study he conducted in Alexandria, Scotland, between 1978 and 1982. Cameron created a database containing the records of every cancer patient attending three hospitals in Scotland during a four-year period. The study found that those cancer patients treated with vitamin C survived for an average of 343 days, versus only 180 days for patients not receiving vitamin C.

Abram Hoffer, M.D., Ph.D., is an internationally respected Canadian doctor who has devoted the last four decades to the field of orthomolecular medicine and the use of niacin (vitamin $B_3$) for treating schizophrenia. Dr. Hoffer has also pioneered the use of vitamin C as a primary agent in his treatment of cancer patients. A paper reporting on Hoffer's work with cancer patients detailed the results of his work between 1990 and 1994. Of the 500 patients who followed Hoffer's nutritional plan, 70 percent were still alive at the end of 1994. By contrast, of the group of 100 patients who did not follow the Hoffer vitamin C plan, only 15 were still alive after four years.

## The Infamous Mayo Study

A study conducted by the Mayo clinic in 1985 made headlines across the world when this prestigious institution announced that their clinical trial, based on the methods of Cameron and Pauling, had failed to find any benefit for vitamin C in cancer patients. Even today, this study, which was led by C. G. Moertel, forms the basis for much of the resistance people encounter when asking their physicians about vitamin C therapy.

For years, vitamin C enthusiasts have pointed out that the Mayo study was seriously flawed and was based on significantly different methods from those described by Pauling and Cameron. These differences prompted researchers from the National Institutes of Health to suggest that the route of administration (intravenous versus oral) may have been the cause of the radically different results.

Intravenous (IV) administration has been shown to result in much higher blood levels of vitamin C than oral administration, and levels that are toxic to certain types of cancer cells in culture can be achieved only with intravenous administration. Part of the problem with understanding what had led to such different outcomes was that Moertel refused to release any information about the study, other than what was in the published paper.

In *Vitamin C & Cancer,* Abram Hoffer revealed the primary reason for the failure of the Mayo study to improve the survival time of cancer patients. In the Mayo therapy, researchers gave 10 g of oral vitamin C per day to a group of fifty patients suffering from advanced colorectal cancer. The significant difference was that, whereas Pauling and Cameron treated patients indefinitely, the Mayo team treated patients only for an average of seventy-five days, and then stopped treatment completely. The result was that as soon as treatment stopped, the patients began to die rapidly. Whereas only one patient died during the seventy-fives days of vitamin C therapy, more than half the patients died within seventy-five days of discontinuing vitamin C.

## Moertel versus Pauling?

The following are some interesting statistics that frequently appear in papers discussing the different viewpoints of Linus Pauling and C. G. Moertel:

**1.** Albert Szent-Györgyi took 1 gram of vitamin C every day and lived to age eighty-nine.

**2.** Linus Pauling consumed 18 g of vitamin C every day and died of prostate cancer at age ninety-four.

**3.** C. G. Moertel of the Mayo Clinic, hostile critic of vitamin C, died of cancer at age sixty-six.

## Antinutrient Bias Exposed

The Mayo study is one of the most blatant examples of the antivitamin bias encountered frequently in medicine and medical research, leading one observer to note that the Mayo study was designed with the "clear intention of blowing the vitamin C and cancer controversy off the medical map." If this is true, it seems to have worked, because every physician has heard about the Mayo study, and based on the published paper, most have formed the opinion that vitamin C is useless in cases of cancer.

## Is Vitamin C Toxic to Cancer Cells?

Preliminary research has recently demonstrated that very high concentrations of vitamin C, in combination with alpha lipoic acid and other natural substances, kills cancer cells outright in laboratory tests. This cytotoxic effect is described as being similar to standard chemotherapy, but with the added benefit of leaving healthy cells undamaged. One of the pioneers in this application of vitamin C is Dr. Hugh Riordan. He has completed a ten-year research project on high-dose intravenous vitamin C and cancer, and his method passed phase I clinical trials at the University of Nebraska Medical School Hospital. These trials established that high-dose vitamin C treatment is nontoxic, and cleared the way for a phase II clinical trial under the auspices of the National Institutes of Health (NIH) for treating renal adenoma (kidney cancer). Dr Riordan has also published several successful case histories, including the results of vitamin C treatment on a late-stage lung cancer patient who remained cancer-free for five years following treatment. This is the generally accepted standard in cancer statistics for a "cure."

## Vitamin C Aids Conventional Cancer Treatment

There has been some question concerning vitamin C's potential to interfere with traditional cancer therapies, including chemotherapy and radiation treatments. Abram Hoffer's addressed this issue, stating, "This [vitamin treatment] would enhance the therapeutic effect of the chemotherapy and decrease its toxicity." Also, " If they [cancer patients] needed chemotherapy the program [vitamin therapy] would make it more tolerable and less painful and if they needed radiation the program would decrease the intensity of the side-effects of the radiation and increase its efficacy."

Proponents of vitamin C therapy recommend that vitamin C should not be used in place of any conventional therapy that has been demonstrated to be effective in the treatment of a particular type of cancer such as chemotherapy or radiation therapy. If an individual with cancer chooses to take vitamin supplements, it is important that the clinician coordinating his or her treatment is aware of the type and dose of each supplement. There is no clinical evidence to suggest that vitamin C has any adverse effect on the survival of cancer patients. However, there is some evidence that the vitamin C treatments should be staggered with the conventional treatments for best results.

# CHAPTER 7

# SAFETY AND POLITICS OF VITAMIN C

Vitamin C has consistently been proven to be an extraordinarily safe nutrient. While a number of possible problems have been raised, most were based on test tube experiments. These concerns include genetic mutations, birth defects, cancer, atherosclerosis, kidney stones, rebound scurvy, increased oxidative stress, excess iron absorption, impaired copper utilization, vitamin $B_{12}$ deficiency, and erosion of dental enamel. In reality, virtually no adverse effects (aside from the laxative effect that can cause loose stools) have been found.

## Kidney Stone Formation

Fears that very high intake of vitamin C could lead to the formation of kidney stones were based on a concern that the production of oxalate, a component of stones that occurs during vitamin C metabolism, would increase stone formation. Research has shown that the oxalate produced from vitamin C is only a fraction of that derived from dietary sources, and there is no safety issue regarding kidney stones.

## Rebound Scurvy

The fear that symptoms of vitamin C deficiency would suddenly appear if large doses of vitamin C were stopped (rebound scurvy) appears to be unfounded in humans, and animal studies with guinea pigs have either shown no such effect, or have been inconclusive.

## Depletion of Vitamin B$_{12}$ and Impaired Copper Absorption

Concerns that large amounts of vitamin C might destroy vitamin B$_{12}$ were found to be the result of errors in experimental testing. Also, controlled studies have found no evidence to support the claim that vitamin C impairs copper absorption.

## Diarrhea

Diarrhea is the only recognized "side effect" that may occur when taking large doses of vitamin C. Unlike diarrhea caused by illness or infection, the loose stools caused by large doses of vitamin C are the first sign that the body's tissue fluids have been saturated with ascorbic acid. This effect is due to the laxative action of vitamin C. Most people will not experience this effect unless they are taking more than 10 g of vitamin C per day. Symptoms are not serious and stop when one either discontinues or reduces the dosage of vitamin C. For more information, see "Dosing to Bowel Tolerance" on page 67.

## Drug Interactions

A number of drugs are known to lower vitamin C levels and may require increased intake of vitamin C. Estrogen-containing contraceptives (birth control pills) are known to lower vitamin C levels in plasma and white blood cells. Aspirin can also lead to lower vitamin C levels if taken frequently. For example, two aspirin tablets taken every six hours for a week have been shown to reduce white blood cell content of vitamin C by 50 percent, primarily by increasing urinary excretion of vitamin C.

# The Politics of Vitamin C

Vitamin C is one of the safest substances known to us. Thousands of studies and research papers support both the clinical effectiveness and exemplary safety record of vitamin C. Yet whenever vitamin C is shown to be useful for any purpose other than simply for preventing scurvy, the antivitamin C lobby can be counted on to quickly produce an "expert" who immediately 1) attacks the findings, 2) questions the methods and/or qualifications of the researchers behind the study, 3) issues warnings against taking any doses greater than the sanctioned RDAs, and 4) calls for further study.

This pattern of doubt and outright hostility is not new—vitamin C and its proponents have been under constant attack for the last several decades. Indeed, hostility to vitamin C goes all the way back to 1746, the year that James Lind proved that scurvy could be prevented with small servings of citrus fruit. The British Navy resisted Lind's findings for forty years in a show of bureaucratic obstinacy that resulted in the deaths of more than 100,000 British sailors.

**Recommended Daily Allowance (RDA)**
*The designated amount of a nutrient needed to prevent overt deficiency disease in most people. RDAs are not enough to promote optimal health or to prevent the incidence of many diseases in all people.*

Part of the hostility toward vitamin C is due to its status as a natural nutrient. Since vitamin C cannot be turned into a patented drug, pharmaceutical companies have no financial incentive to perform the double-blind studies that most of the scientific community need to be convinced of a substance's effectiveness.

Additionally, because of the seriousness of cancer and the political environment within the medical system, the use of vitamin C to prevent or treat cancer is a highly charged and controversial issue with conventional physicians.

## The Attack on Vitamin C

In one recent attack, a letter published in the April 9, 1998 issue of *Nature* outlined claims by a group of British researchers who suggested that 500 mg of vitamin C per day could cause damage to human DNA. The media responded to what was essentially a press release with a flood of alarming reports stating that vitamin C caused cancer. Subsequent research found these conclusions to be entirely wrong, concluding that supplementing with 500 mg of vitamin C per day and 400 IU of vitamin E had "no significant main effect or interaction effect on oxidative DNA damage." Unfortunately, when this report was published, the mainstream press failed to share the information with the public.

The letter published in *Nature* was followed two years later by a report published in the journal *Science,* which stated that lipid hydroperoxides (rancid fat molecules) can react with vitamin C in a test tube to form products that are potentially harmful to DNA. Although the reaction of these products with DNA was not demonstrated in the study, it was suggested that vitamin C might enhance mutations and increase the risk of cancer. That this conclusion was unwarranted and contradicted countless studies showing vitamin C's benefits did little to stop the media from churning out a new rash of alarming headlines implying that vitamin C caused cancer.

## Flawed Science

One of the biggest problems with the study reported in *Science* was that it tested conditions that simply do not exist in the real world. In living cells, vitamin C acts as the first line of antioxidant defense, directly preventing the formation of lipid hydroperoxides. In fact, lipid hydroperoxides can form only when vitamin C levels have been depleted. Vitamin C also works in conjunction with vitamin E—both antioxidants recycle each other to quench free radicals. Additionally, vitamin E also provides additional defense by directly preventing the conversion of unsaturated fats to lipid hydroperoxides. When (and if) lipid hydroperoxides do occur in the body, a number of cellular enzymes go to work to instantly reduce these compounds into harmless alcohols. In the study in question, researchers incubated vitamin C in concentrations of lipid hydroperoxides at least 10,000 times higher than could possibly exist in human plasma, for time periods of up to two hours—far longer than the fraction of a second it would take before enzymes rendered them harmless.

## Consumer Awareness

Vitamin C supplements are often singled out as potential troublemakers, though the body does not distinguish between dietary vitamin C and supplemental vitamin C. Thus, if vitamin C indeed caused cancer, as some antinutrient doctors have suggested, the only advice one could follow would be to stop taking vitamin supplements while also eliminating vitamin C–rich fruits and vegetables from the diet! In reality, we know that vitamin C–rich foods lower the risk of cancer, heart disease, stroke, and other diseases, so the more fruits and vegetables you eat, the better.

## Media Bias versus Scientific Fact

While the findings reported in *Science* turned out to have little relevance to the actual processes that occur in human beings, the manner in which the story was handled revealed much about the media bias against supplements. Contemporary media is a competitive business that is driven by immediacy and sensationalism. And American media often reveals an "antisupplement" tendency in its uncritical acceptance of any report touting the potential dangers of nutrients. To support their more sensational headlines, news outlets tend to interview conventional doctors and scientist who remain steadfast in their unwillingness to accept that vitamins and minerals might have health benefits, while refusing to include opposing viewpoints.

In 1999, Dr. Hoffer summed up the problem nicely when, writing about the reluctance of orthodox physicians to accept the scientific evidence on the safety of vitamin C, he stated: "They will still promote their old ideas and will bolster them by manufacturing toxicities. As a rule, when there are no toxicities, it is simple to invent them, such as vitamin C causes kidney stones, or damages the liver, or interferes with the treatment of diabetes and so on. Every month I hear about new toxicities which totally surprise and delight me because they indicate how imaginative my colleagues can be."

# CHAPTER 8

# How Much Vitamin C Should You Take?

Following publication of Linus Pauling's *Vitamin C and the Common Cold* in 1970, consumption of vitamin C in the United States shot up by more than 300 percent. Average intake of vitamin C continues to grow each year, and for good reason. A recent study determined that vitamin C blood levels are a good predictor of mortality risk. Higher blood levels of vitamin C have been shown to indicate a lower risk for developing cardiovascular diseases and certain types of cancer and degenerative diseases. In this chapter, we'll review the most common standards and recommendations for vitamin C dosages.

## Recommended Daily Allowance of Vitamin C

Many people still base their vitamin C intake on the recommended daily allowance (RDA). This is unfortunate because, while these amounts certainly protect against outright scurvy in most people, they fall far below the minimal levels currently shown to prevent many chronic and age-related degenerative conditions associated with long-term, low-level vitamin C deficiency. Despite evidence that higher vitamin C intake will enhance health and decrease the incidence of disease, political considerations have delayed attempts to raise the RDA for decades.

Recently, the RDA for vitamin C has been revised upward from 60 mg daily to 75 mg per day for women, and 90 mg per day for men. The recommended intake for smokers is 35 mg per day higher than for nonsmokers, because smokers are under increased oxidative stress from the toxins in cigarette smoke and generally have lower blood levels of vitamin C.

## The Problem with RDAs

Today, many researchers and scientists recommend raising the RDA even higher, to a minimum of 200 mg per day, based on the current understanding of the vital role vitamin C plays in promoting health. Furthermore, even a dosage of 200 mg per day would not be enough to address the higher vitamin C requirements of women, children, middle aged and elderly adults, and individuals dealing with special circumstances (special

| TABLE 8.1. Recommended Dietary Allowance (RDA) for Vitamin C | | | |
|---|---|---|---|
| Life Stage | Age | Men (mg/day) | Women (mg/day) |
| Children | 1–3 | 15 | 15 |
| Children | 4–8 | 25 | 25 |
| Children | 9–13 | 45 | 45 |
| Adolescents | 14–18 | 75 | 65 |
| Adults | 19 and over | 90 | 75 |
| Smokers | 19 and over | 125 | 110 |
| Pregnancy | 18 and under | — | 80 |
| Pregnancy | 19 and over | — | 85 |
| Breastfeeding | 18 and under | — | 115 |
| Breastfeeding | 19 and over | — | 120 |

diets, tobacco smoking, sickness, infections, trauma, metabolic and genetic disorders, or degenerative diseases).

## Vitamin C for Optimal Health

Based on the overwhelmingly positive reports on the benefits of higher levels of vitamin C, many nutritionally based physicians now recommend that people base their intake of vitamin C on how much they need to promote *optimal health*, not just to prevent scurvy.

Taking a cue from animals still able to produce their own vitamin C, researchers have examined the levels produced by various species, seeking clues to help determine just how much vitamin C humans might need to maintain optimal health.

Remember that all animals, apart from primates and guinea pigs, are able to manufacture vitamin C in their livers. And while the amount produced is different in each species, every single animal produces vitamin C in levels that are hundreds, if not thousands, of times higher than those required to simply prevent scurvy. This is puzzling when one considers that glucose, which is used to make vitamin C, is absolutely vital for energy production.

Nature does not design for waste, and depleting glucose levels—and potentially running out of energy at a crucial point—can mean the difference between life and death in the constant battle for survival. The reasonable answer for these extraordinarily high levels of vitamin C, produced at the cost of life-giving glucose, is that they are essential for the health and survival of these animals.

Table 8.2 lists the average amount of vitamin C produced by each animal in the left column. In the right column, we see the equivalent amount of vitamin C, as extrapolated to the body weight of a 154-pound human. As you can see, if humans had

**TABLE 8.2.**
## Average Amount of Vitamin C Produced by Animals and the Human Equivalent

| Animal | Vitamin C | Vitamin C equivalent produced per day for 154-pound human |
|--------|-----------|-----------------------------------------------------------|
| Cat | 336 mg | 2,800 mg |
| Cow | 1,099 mg | 1,281 mg |
| Goat | 2,280 mg | 13,300 mg |
| Mouse | 2,352 mg | 19,250 mg |
| Rabbit | 1,547 mg | 15,820 mg |
| Rat | 2,737 mg | 13,902 mg |

not lost their ability to manufacture vitamin C—a loss that many now view as a genetic disease—our daily production of vitamin C would likely be between 3,000 and 15,000 mg per day, or an average of 5,400 mg per day under normal (healthy) circumstances. Research has also shown that some animals, when their health is under stress, are not always able to produce enough vitamin C. Cats and dogs, for example, are relatively low vitamin C producers, and are susceptible to stress-related vitamin C deficiency.

## Optimal Doses for Humans

So what does this mean for you, and what can be considered a safe dose of vitamin C for optimal health? Recommendations differ widely, depending on the source. While many traditional doctors might feel uncomfortable about openly recommending vitamin C in doses higher than the RDAs, a recent survey in the United States found that those doctors who are the healthiest report that they consume on average at least 250 mg of vitamin C per day. Many health professionals admit to taking even higher doses.

Many holistic and alternative medical researchers suggest that, based on countless medical studies, a more reasonable therapeutic intake of vitamin C would range from 500–4,000 mg per day. This water-soluble vitamin is completely excreted from the body within four hours under normal circumstances. To maintain stable serum levels, the desired total daily dose should be divided into three separate doses taken throughout the day.

## Dosing to Bowel Tolerance

Ask a vitamin C expert like Dr. Robert Cathcart how much vitamin C to take, and the answer is likely to be "a lot." Dr. Cathcart has long recommended the "bowel tolerance" method of determining one's need. This is determined by taking increasingly large amounts of vitamin C each day until your body reaches the saturation point. Any amount beyond that level and vitamin C becomes a laxative. Based on his experience with more than 20,000 patients, Dr. Cathcart believes that the bowel tolerance level for most healthy people is between 10–15 g of vitamin C per day. When fighting a cold or flu, bowel tolerance rises to between 30–60 g, and for those with a serious infectious illness, the need to induce tolerance can jump to 200 g per day or more. During an infectious illness, the best clinical results have been achieved by maintaining high vitamin C levels in the blood by taking 3 g or more of vitamin C every four hours.

When Dr. Cathcart treated patients for mononucleosis, most were functioning normally after a few days of receiving 200 g of vitamin C per day, given orally and intravenously. This was in sharp contrast to other patients in the same community, who were often hospitalized for several weeks during a mononucleosis outbreak.

## Is Vitamin C "Expensive Urine"?

One of the most frequent charges made against taking vitamin C in high doses is, that since much of the vitamin is excreted within a matter of hours, all one is doing is making "expensive urine." Researchers investigated this by giving increasingly larger daily doses and measuring excretion in the urine to see how much was needed to saturate tissue levels. They found that only a quarter of the subjects reached their vitamin C maximum at 1,500 mg a day. More than half of those in the study required more than 2,500 mg a day to reach a level where their bodies could use no more. In several cases, test subjects did not reach their maximum even at 5,000 mg per day!

Another consideration, pointed out by Dr. Michael Colgan, an internationally renowned nutritional research scientist, is that vitamin C protects the bowel, kidneys, and bladder as it exits the body. This is an added bonus, since the average victim of bowel or bladder cancer, aside from their pain and suffering, spends $26,000 for treatment—mostly to no avail.

Another way to look at vitamin C excretion is by thinking of what it takes to put out a house fire. The only solution is to pour as much water on the flames, as fast as possible, to put out the fire and save the house. There is little concern about "saving" the water used in this process, and no one cares that, after quenching the flames, the excess water just evaporates or drains away. The value of water in this case is not the water itself, but what the water can do to contribute to putting out the flames and saving lives. In much the same way, optimal health is not about "losing value" when vitamin C is eventually excreted, but in "getting value" by using it in high enough doses, and maintaining serum levels long enough, to quench the free-radical fires damaging our bodies.

Dr. Cathcart uses a similar analogy when describing how megadose vitamin C therapy works. "Suppose you owned a farm and on one end of the property there was a barn and on the other end of the property there was a water well. One day the barn catches fire and neighbors come with buckets to set up a bucket brigade between the water well and the barn and are putting out the fire when the well goes dry.

My use of vitamin C is like thousands of neighbors coming from miles around, each with a bucketful of their own water, throwing their own water on your fire once, and then leaving."

## Vitamin C for Disease Prevention

As we've seen, the amount of vitamin C required for chronic diseases is much higher than that required simply to prevent scurvy. Much of the information regarding vitamin C and the prevention of chronic disease is based on studies that measure vitamin C intake in large groups of people, over periods of years or decades, to determine a protective effect against chronic diseases. The following list describes vitamin C doses discussed in research studies conducted across the globe over the last thirty years. While not recommendations, the amounts described may serve as guidance in researching and determining your own need for vitamin C.

## Age-Related Memory Impairment

Antioxidant blood levels have been shown to improve memory performance in the elderly. Higher vitamin C blood levels are associated with significant improvements in recognition, vocabulary, and memory recall. Doses of 500–1,000 mg per day have been used for this condition.

## Allergies (Hay Fever)

Vitamin C is a natural antihistamine that has been shown to help suppress allergic reactions. Doses of 2,000–12,000 mg per day have been used for this condition.

## Alzheimer's Disease

Researchers have shown that people with Alzheimer's disease have lower blood levels of vitamin C. When given 1,000 mg of vitamin C per day, blood levels increased significantly in people with Alzheimer's disease. In a study of vitamin C intake, out of 633 people aged sixty-five and older, 91 developed Alzheimer's disease over a period of four and a quarter years, but none of the 23 vitamin C supplement users developed the condition. Doses of 1,000–2,000 mg per day have been used for this condition.

## Angina Pectoris

Vitamin C has been shown to improve blood vessel dilation that is often compromised in people with atherosclerosis. The pain of angina pectoris is also related to impaired dilation of the coronary arteries. Treatment with 500 mg per day of vitamin C has been proven to improve dilation of blood vessels in individuals with angina pectoris and congestive heart failure. Doses of 500–1,000 mg per day have been used for this condition.

## Osteoarthritis and Rheumatoid Arthritis

Vitamin C has been shown effective in helping to reduce the progression of arthritis. A dosage of

420 mg of vitamin C per day resulted in a 300 percent reduction in the progression of the disease and reduced joint pain, particularly in the knees. Researchers have also shown that blood levels of vitamin C are extremely low in patients with rheumatoid arthritis, suggesting that vitamin C may offer antioxidant protection to reduce damage to inflamed joints. Doses of 420–2,000 mg per day have been used for these conditions.

## Asthma

Vitamin C is helpful in the treatment of asthma, particularly in patients with food allergies. Histamine is a major factor in asthmatic attacks, and vitamin C is proven to speed up the natural clearing of excess histamine in the serum. Asthmatics can take 2 g or more of vitamin C to help break down mucus involved in attacks. Taken at bedtime, 500–1000 mg of vitamin C has been shown to reduce or prevent asthma attacks that occur in the middle of the night. Doses of 2,000–5,000 mg per day have been used for this condition.

## Diabetes

Numerous studies have shown that vitamin C plasma levels are about 30 percent lower in people with diabetes, as compared with people who do not have diabetes. In one study, researchers found that high doses of vitamin C markedly improved blood-sugar regulation in people with non–insulin-dependent diabetes mellitus (NIDDM). Vitamin C has also been shown to improve blood vessel dilation, which is often impaired in people with diabetes.

**Diabetes Epidemic**
*Diabetes has increased 49 percent from 1990 to 2000, and NIH projections indicate a 165 percent increase by the year 2050!*

Also, complications of diabetes are linked to increased oxidative stresses, supporting a role for vitamin C in preventing some of the complications of diabetes. Vitamin C helps to reduce the abnormal attachment of sugars to proteins (glycosylation). Doses of between 100 and 600 mg of vitamin C per day have been shown to normalize cellular sorbitol levels, which may have implications for decreasing some of the long-term complications of diabetes. Doses of 500–1,000 mg per day have been used for this condition.

**Glycosylation**
*A process that binds sugars (glucose) with proteins in the body to form dangerous compounds that complicate aging and diabetes.*

## Cancer

Vitamin C has been proven to protect against a number of types of cancer in doses as low as 100–500 mg per day. Additionally, Pauling and Cameron found that dosages of 10 g per day improved both the survival time and the quality of life of terminal cancer patients. Research has shown that high blood levels of vitamin C are toxic to certain types of cancers, and such levels can be achieved only by (IV) administration, as was initially used in the Pauling/Cameron study. Doses of 10,000–100,000 mg per day have been used for this condition.

## Cataracts

Decreased vitamin C levels in the lens of the eye are linked to cataracts in humans. Several studies have shown that increased intake of vitamin C may decrease the incidence of cataracts. Researchers have shown that a daily dose of 300 mg of vitamin C has a protective effect against the development of cataracts when taken for a number of years. Doses of 300–500 mg per day have been used for this condition.

## Gingivitis

Low levels of vitamin C are often associated with gingivitis. Doses of 500–4,000 mg of vitamin C per day have been shown to improve gum conditions.

## Glaucoma

Vitamin C reduces elevated intraocular pressure (IOP) in the eye by helping fluid exit the eye and flow into the blood. Vitamin C also diminishes the production of eye fluid and improves fluid outflow. Vitamin C must be taken in large doses—between 20 and 35 g per day. Vitamin C therapy is not a cure, and if intake is reduced or stopped, glaucoma will continue to develop at its previous pace. Doses of 5,000–35,000 mg per day have been used for this condition.

## Hepatitis

Reports from German literature show that high doses of vitamin C are beneficial in treating epidemic hepatitis in children. Doses of 2 g of vitamin C per day have been shown to stimulate the immune response and help to fight infection. Beneficial effects were also observed in sixty-three cases of epidemic hepatitis treated with 10 g of vitamin C daily for an average of five days. The patients' hospital stays and symptoms were reduced by 50 percent. Doses of 5,000–10,000 mg per day have been used for this condition.

## HIV

Vitamin C acts as an antiviral agent, elevating the body's interferon levels. Vitamin C has also been found to inhibit HIV replication in laboratory tests. Bowel tolerance with vitamin C is recommended for its antioxidant and immunity-enhancing abilities and to increase disease resistance and improve well-being in patients with HIV. Doses of

5,000–20,000 mg per day have been used for this condition.

## Hypertension (High Blood Pressure)

Several studies have shown that supplemental vitamin C can have a blood pressure–lowering effect. In a recent study, as little as 500 mg of vitamin C per day resulted in an average drop in systolic blood pressure of 9 percent after four weeks. Doses of 6,000 mg per day have been used for this condition.

## Influenza

Vitamin C has been shown to help prevent flu infection, and when taken in high doses, it speeds recovery from influenza. Doses of 2,000–6,000 mg per day have been used for this condition.

## Lead Poisoning

Lead poisoning continues to be a significant health problem in the United States, especially for children living in urban areas. Children exposed to lead are more likely to develop learning disabilities and behavioral problems and to have low IQs. Abnormal growth and development have also been observed in children born to women exposed to lead during pregnancy. Several studies have shown that low intake of vitamin C is associated with higher blood levels of lead. Research suggests that vitamin C protects against lead poisoning by inhibiting intestinal absorption while enhancing urinary excretion of lead, significantly lowering blood lead levels in as little as four weeks. Doses of 1,000–2,000 mg per day have been used for this condition.

## Macular Degeneration

Antioxidants have been shown to prevent the oxidative damage that causes macular degeneration.

People with high blood levels of vitamin C and other antioxidants, such as vitamin E and selenium, have a 70 percent lower risk of developing macular degeneration. Doses of 500–1,000 mg per day have been used for this condition.

## Male Infertility

Vitamin C protects sperm from oxidative damage, and improves sperm quality, particularly in smokers. Taking 1 g of vitamin C per day has also been found effective in treating sperm agglutination, a condition that causes sperm to clump together. Doses of 1,000–2,000 mg per day have been used for this condition.

## Retinopathy

Antioxidants have been shown to prevent the oxidative damage that causes retinopathy. Vitamin C also strengthens the capillaries that supply blood to the retina. Vitamin C and other antioxidants, such as vitamin E and selenium, have been shown to reduce the damaging effects of retinopathy. Doses of 500–2,000 mg per day have been used for this condition.

## Schizophrenia

In 1966, researchers showed that adult men with schizophrenia required 36–48 g of vitamin C per day to reach the vitamin C saturation level that normal men reach with only 4 g of vitamin C per day. While the patients were by no means cured, the high doses of vitamin C brought about marked improvement in the socialization of the patients. Those who were shy, reclusive, and withdrawn began to participate in ward activities and in conversation with other patients and ward personnel. Doses of 36,000–48,000 mg per day have been used for this condition.

# CHAPTER 9

# FORMS OF VITAMIN C

When deciding which form of vitamin C is best, keep in mind that, as Linus Pauling pointed out, all forms of vitamin C are identical. The body doesn't care if the C is "natural" or synthesized, just as long as it gets enough of it. True, there are some benefits to natural food sources of C, such as fruits and vegetables. They can provide other nutrients, such as bioflavonoids. On the other hand, supplements have the advantage of packing a lot of vitamin C into a very small serving. You would have to drink eight glasses of orange juice, eat sixteen oranges, or consume fifty cups of blueberries to equal the vitamin C found in one 1,000-mg capsule. In short, when choosing your vitamin C, the most important point is choosing a form that agrees with your lifestyle and your budget.

## Getting Vitamin C from Foods

Vitamin C can be obtained in various amounts from food sources, primarily from fruits and vegetables. As shown in Table 9.1 below, fruits and vegetables vary in their vitamin C content, but five servings should average out to at least 200 mg of vitamin C. Vitamin C is easily destroyed by heat, and because it is water-soluble, this vitamin can be drained off in liquids used in food preparation. To assure full potency of vitamin C value, it is best to consume foods raw or minimally processed.

## TABLE 9.1.
# Good Food Sources of Vitamin C

| Food/<br>Serving Size | Vitamin C<br>Content |
|---|---|
| Fresh Orange Juice, 1 cup | 124 mg |
| Green Pepper, 1/2 cup | 96 mg |
| Grapefruit Juice, 1 cup | 93 mg |
| Papaya, 1/2 medium | 85 mg |
| Brussels Sprouts, 4 medium | 73 mg |
| Broccoli, raw, 1/2 cup | 70 mg |
| Orange, 1 medium | 66 mg |
| Cantaloupe, 1/4 medium | 45 mg |
| Cauliflower, 1/2 cup | 45 mg |
| Strawberries, 1/2 cup | 44 mg |
| Tomato Juice, 1 cup | 39 mg |
| Cabbage, 1/2 cup | 21 mg |
| Blackberries, 1/2 cup | 15 mg |
| Spinach, raw, 1/2 cup | 14 mg |
| Blueberries, 1/2 cup | 10 mg |
| Cherries, 1/2 cup | 8 mg |

**Note:** *Values given are estimates derived from the USDA Nutrient Values database.*

## Getting Your Vitamin C from Supplements

Vitamin C supplements are available in many forms, but according to the Linus Pauling Institute, there is little scientific evidence to show that any one form is better absorbed or more effective than another.

Natural and synthetic forms of vitamin C are chemically identical, and there are no known differences in their biological activity. The possibility that vitamin C from natural sources might be more bioavailable than synthetic vitamin C has been investigated in at least two human studies and no significant differences were found.

Mineral salts of vitamin C are buffered and are, therefore, less acidic than ascorbic acid. Some people find them less irritating to the gastrointestinal tract than ascorbic acid. Sodium ascorbate and calcium ascorbate are the most common forms, although a number of other mineral ascorbates are available. Sodium ascorbate generally provides 131 mg of sodium per 1,000 mg of ascorbic acid, and pure calcium ascorbate provides 114 mg of calcium per 1,000 mg of ascorbic acid.

Buffered vitamin C powder is prepared from beets (virtually all other forms are derived from corn). Because buffered vitamin C has an acid-alkaline buffering action, it can help control the increased acidity often associated with allergic reactions. Many of the most severely ill, allergic, or hypersensitive people can tolerate buffered C, even when unable to tolerate other vitamin C products.

Bioflavonoids are water-soluble plant pigments that are often found in vitamin C–rich fruits and vegetables, especially citrus fruit. Vitamin C activity is enhanced when taken with natural bioflavonoids, such as hesperidin and rutin.

Ascorbyl palmitate is a fat-soluble form of vitamin C that protects fats from peroxidation. Ascorbyl palmitate can be stored in the body in small amounts. Ascorbyl palmitate has been added to a number of skin creams due to its antioxidant properties and the role of vitamin C in collagen synthesis.

# CONCLUSION

**M**illions of years ago, a genetic accident impaired our ability to produce vitamin C, a basic requirement for life. If not for this ancient genetic accident, humans today would normally produce vitamin C in levels measured in tens of grams per day. Evidence suggests that restoring vitamin C to higher levels would benefit modern human health and reduce the incidence of degenerative and infectious diseases, fend off the effects of old age, and endow all with longer lives.

Today, vitamin C is becoming one of the most widely used and valued vitamins due to its ability to help humans correct our inherited genetic defect. In addition to being the safest vitamin known to us, we have seen how the vast array of important health benefits of vitamin C improve health and prolong life by:

1. Acting as a powerful, water-soluble antioxidant to protect us against free radicals. Vitamin C has also been proven to save lives by reducing the oxidative damage that causes atherosclerosis.

2. Producing healthy collagen and strong connective tissues to keep muscles, blood vessels, bones, and teeth young and healthy.

3. Helping the body use other vital nutrients, such as folic acid (for maintaining healthy

DNA) and iron (for hemoglobin, the oxygen-carrying part of blood cells).

4.  Aiding the synthesis of neurotransmitters that energize us, help us sleep, control aches and pains, and maintain a positive mood.

5.  Supporting the immune system in the constant battle against cancer, infections, and the degenerative diseases common to aging.

6.  Increasing formation of liver bile to aid in the removal of cholesterol and potentially toxic substances, such as lead.

7.  Helping to transport and burn fats and carbohydrates in the mitochondria for energy.

8.  Keeping blood vessels and arteries open and dilated to prevent arterial spasms and heart attacks.

9.  Maintaining antioxidant levels in the eyes to prevent macular degeneration and cataracts.

10. Protecting people with diabetes from the damage caused by increased levels of sorbitol in the bloodstream.

We hope that this brief overview of vitamin C has conveyed some of the power and importance of this essential antiaging, anticancer, and anti-stress nutrient. Hopefully we have conveyed the very real message, that—whether you get your vitamin C from fruits and vegetables, or high-potency vitamins—the evidence proves that you can expect to live a longer, healthier, and more fulfilling life.

# SELECTED
# REFERENCES

Cameron E, Pauling L. Supplemental ascorbate in the supportive treatment of cancer: Prolongation of survival times in terminal human cancer. *Proceedings of the National Academy of Science, USA,* 1976; 73(10):3685–3689.

Carr AC, Frei B. Toward a new recommended dietary allowance for vitamin C based on antioxidant and health effects in humans. *American Journal of Clinical Nutrition,* 1999;69(6):1086–1107.

Cheng Y, Willett WC, Schwartz J, et al. Relation of nutrition to bone lead and blood lead levels in middle-aged to elderly men. The Normative Aging Study. *American Journal of Epidemiology,* 1998; 147(12):1162–1174.

DeRitter E. Physiologic availability of dehydro-L-ascorbic acid and palmitoyl-L-ascorbic acid. *Science,* 1951;113:628–631.

Duffy SJ, Gokce N, Holbrook M, et al. Treatment of hypertension with ascorbic acid. *Lancet,* 1999;354 (9195):2048–2049.

Food and Nutrition Board, Institute of Medicine. Vitamin C. Dietary Reference Intakes for Vitamin C, Vitamin E, Selenium, and Carotenoids. Washington D.C.: National Academy Press; 2000:95–185.

Gokce N, Keaney JF, Jr., Frei B, et al. Long-term ascorbic acid administration reverses endothelial vasomotor dysfunction in patients with coronary artery disease. *Circulation,* 1999;99(25):3234–3240.

Hemila H. Vitamin C intake and susceptibility to the common cold. *British Journal of Nutrition,* 1997; 77(1):59–72.

Jacques PF, Chylack LT, Jr., Hankinson SE, et al. Long-term nutrient intake and early age-related nuclear lens opacities. *Archives of Ophthalmology,* 2001; 119(7):1009–1019.

Khaw KT, Bingham S, Welch A, et al. Relation between plasma ascorbic acid and mortality in men and women in EPIC-Norfolk prospective study: A prospective population study. European Prospective Investigation into Cancer and Nutrition. *Lancet,* 2001;357(9257):657–663.

Kromhout D. Essential micronutrients in relation to carcinogenesis. *American Journal of Clinical Nutrition,* 1987;45(5 Suppl):1361–1367.

Lee SH, Oe T, Blair IA. Vitamin C-induced decomposition of lipid hydroperoxides to endogenous genotoxins. *Science,* 2001;292(5524):2083–2086.

Levine M, Rumsey SC, Daruwala R, Park JB, Wang Y. Criteria and recommendations for vitamin C intake. *Journal of the American Medical Association,* 1999; 281(15):1415–1423.

Michels KB, Holmberg L, Bergkvist L, Ljung H, Bruce A, Wolk A. Dietary antioxidant vitamins, retinol, and breast cancer incidence in a cohort of Swedish women. *International Journal of Cancer,* 2001;91(4): 563–567.

Moertel CG, Fleming TR, Creagan ET, Rubin J, O'-Connell MJ, Ames MM. High-dose vitamin C versus placebo in the treatment of patients with advanced cancer who have had no prior chemotherapy. A randomized double-blind comparison. *New England Journal of Medicine,* 1985;312(3):137–141.

Padayatty SJ, Levine M. Reevaluation of ascorbate in cancer treatment: Emerging evidence, open minds and serendipity. *Journal of the American College of Nutrition*, 2000;19(4):423–425.

Sauberlich, HE. A history of scurvy and vitamin C. In Packer, L. and Fuchs, J. Eds. *Vitamin C in Health and Disease*. New York: Marcel Decker Inc., 1997: pp. 1–24.

Simon JA, Hudes ES. Relationship of ascorbic acid to blood lead levels. *Journal of the American Medical Association*, 1999;281(24):2289–2293.

Simon JA, Hudes ES. Serum ascorbic acid and gall-bladder disease prevalence among US adults: The Third National Health and Nutrition Examination Survey (NHANES III). *Archives of Internal Medicine*, 2000;160(7):931–936.

Steinmetz KA, Potter JD. Vegetables, fruit, and cancer prevention: a review. *Journal of the American Dietetic Association*, 1996;96(10):1027–1039.

Weinstein M, Babyn P, Zlotkin S. An orange a day keeps the doctor away: Scurvy in the year 2000. *Pediatrics*, 2001;108(3):E55.

Will JC, Byers T. Does diabetes mellitus increase the requirement for vitamin C? *Nutrition Review*, 1996; 54(7):193–202.

Will JC, Ford ES, Bowman BA. Serum vitamin C concentrations and diabetes: Findings from the Third National Health and Nutrition Examination Survey, 1988–1994. *American Journal of Clinical Nutrition*, 1999;70(1):49–52.

Yokoyama T, Date C, Kokubo Y, Yoshiike N, Matsumura Y, Tanaka H. Serum vitamin C concentration was inversely associated with subsequent 20-year incidence of stroke in a Japanese rural community. The Shibata Study. *Stroke, 2000;31(10): 2287–2294.*

# OTHER BOOKS
# AND RESOURCES

Cameron, Ewan, Linus Pauling (Contributor). *Cancer and Vitamin C: A Discussion of the Nature, Causes, Prevention, and Treatment of Cancer.* Philadelphia, PA: Camino Books, 1993.

Cheraskin, E. *Vitamin C: Who Needs It?* Brooklyn, NY: Arlington Press, 1993.

Packer, Lester, and Jurgen Fuchs (eds.). *Vitamin C in Health and Disease.* New York, NY: Marcel Dekker, Inc., 1997.

Pauling, Dr. Linus. *How to Live Longer and Feel Better,* Reissue Edition. New York, NY: Avon, 1996.

Stone, Irwin. *The Healing Factor: "Vitamin C" Against Disease.* New York, NY: Putnam Publishing Group, 1974.

### GreatLife Magazine
Consumer magazine with articles on vitamins, minerals, herbs, and foods.
*Available for free at many health and natural food stores.*

### Let's Live Magazine
Consumer magazine with emphasis on the health benefits of vitamins, minerals, and herbs.
Customer service:
1-800-676-4333

P.O. Box 74908
Los Angeles, CA 90004
*Subscriptions: 12 issues per year, $19.95 in the U.S.;*
*$31.95 outside the U.S.*

### Physical Magazine
Magazine oriented to body builders and other serious athletes.

Customer service:
1-800-676-4333
P.O. Box 74908
Los Angeles, CA 90004
*Subscriptions: 12 issues per year, $19.95 in the U.S.;*
*$31.95 outside the U.S.*

### The Nutrition Reporter™ newsletter
Monthly newsletter that summarizes recent medical research on vitamins, minerals, and herbs.

Customer service:
P.O. Box 30246
Tucson, AZ 85751-0246
e-mail: jack@thenutritionreporter.com
www.nutritionreporter.com
*Subscriptions: $26 per year (12 issues) in the U.S.; $32*
*U.S. or $48 CNC for Canada; $38 for other countries*

## WEBSITES

C For Yourself
http://www.cforyourself.com

The Linus Pauling Institute
http://www.orst.edu/dept/lpi/

Orthomolecular Oncology
http://www.canceraction.org.gg/diff.htm

Vitamin C: Orthomolecular Medicine website
http://www.orthomed.com

# INDEX

# BASIC HEALTH PUBLICATIONS USER'S GUIDES TO NUTRITIONAL SUPPLEMENTS

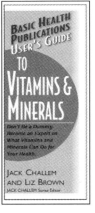

## USER'S GUIDE TO VITAMINS & MINERALS

**Jack Challem & Liz Brown**

Are vitamins really good for you? How about minerals? Thousands of scientific studies say definitely! Vitamins and minerals are required for every aspect of your health—your heart, resistance to infection and cancer, and even for thinking clearly. The *User's Guide to Vitamins & Minerals* explains how these remarkable nutrients can make a big difference in your health.

**About the Authors:** Jack Challem, a leading American health writer, is editor of *The Nutrition Reporter*™ newsletter (www.nutritionreporter.com) and principal author of *Syndrome X: The Complete Nutrition Program to Prevent and Reverse Insulin Resistance.* His scientific articles have appeared in *Medical Hypotheses, Free Radical Biology and Medicine,* and the *Journal of the National Cancer Institute.* He is also editor for the User's Guide to Nutritional Supplements Series.

Liz Brown is a freelance health and nutrition writer based in Portland, Oregon. She earned a B.S. in Nutrition from the University of Minnesota–Twin Cities and regularly contributes articles to various magazines and newspapers.

*ISBN: 1-59120-004-0 • 96 pages • 3.75" x 8.5"*
*Health/Nutrition • $5.95/Can. $9.50*